The Small-Boat Skipper's
SAFETY BOOK

DENNY DESOUTTER

The Small-Boat Skipper's
SAFETY BOOK

Illustrations by
DAVID JENKINS

HOLLIS & CARTER

LONDON SYDNEY

TORONTO

© Denny Desoutter 1972, 1977
Paperback edition ISBN 0 370 30011 4
Hard-cover edition ISBN 0 370 30010 6
Printed Offset Litho in Great Britain for
Hollis & Carter
an associate company of
The Bodley Head Ltd
9 Bow Street, London WC2E 7AL
by Cox & Wyman Ltd, Fakenham
Set in Monotype Imprint
First published 1972
Reprinted 1973
*Second edition, revised, first
published as a paperback and
simultaneously in hard covers 1977*

CONTENTS

INTRODUCTION

The Cry in the Night

'Quiet a minute – what was that . . . I thought I heard someone call.'

I rested on my oars to listen. It was a black night, late, and the creek seemed deserted as we pulled towards our mooring. A faint light glowed from a moored boat downstream, but even the quay where we had loaded our weekend stores into the dinghy was now lost in the darkness astern. We had been feeling our way by the silhouettes of the trees along the shore, and the occasional shadowy shape of a familiar boat, or her mast against the sky.

Drifting, we listened to the drip of the water from the oars, and then there was no mistaking it – a call for help from somewhere downstream.

'Down that way, I think,' said Dorothy. 'By that boat with the light.'

I rowed, she fished in her handbag for the torch. A few strokes, then rest and listen. 'Ahoy, we're coming – keep calling.'

And call he certainly did. With help on its way he wasn't going to miss his chance. We found him downstream of the lighted boat, clinging to a mooring buoy, still fit, but cold and with good reason to be worried for the tide was running seaward at about 4 knots. How we got him into our dinghy (which was not easy) and safely back to his boat is not a matter of immediate concern. Nor is the astonishment of a wife who saw a soaking wet husband step down to the cabin on a night when it was not raining. What is of importance is that one man came near to his death because he was careless enough to fall overboard. And what happened to him could happen to anyone.

Like so many owner-skippers, he was in the habit of going on deck for a last look round before bedtime. 'It was so silly,' he said. 'I had left the ensign up, and as I stepped up to the after deck from the cockpit I caught one foot under the tiller and rolled quite comfortably into the water. I almost saved myself, but my fingers slipped from the toerail, and there I was going downstream at a rate of knots. With all my clothes on I couldn't make headway back to the boat, so rather than struggle fruitlessly I thought it would be better to make across the stream, towards the shore.'

But even that had proved too tiring, and when he saw a mooring buoy he was glad of the chance to hang on. His dinghy, an inflatable, was on deck, and not lying astern where it might have served as 'long stop' so to speak. His wife, listening drowsily to the radio in the cabin would sooner or later have wondered why he was so long on deck. But would she have been able to get the rubber dinghy overboard herself, and would it have been soon enough? A man does not last long in cold water, and a matter of ten minutes more could have turned a wetting into a drowning, even though it might seem unbelievable that a strong, experienced yachtsman could drown from a well-found boat lying peacefully at her mooring on a calm May night.

When he had dried and changed, we sat in their cabin, helping him enjoy his medicinal Scotch, and talked about the *silly* and needless accidents we had suffered, or seen, or heard of. On one thing we were all agreed; that many of the 'dangers of the sea' have their origins in very trivial causes, and that it takes a lively imagination to foresee the train of events that may end in disaster.

I forbore to mention it at that time, but I pictured to myself the further danger to that man's wife had she found he was missing and tried to launch the dinghy from the deck. Working hastily, perhaps a bit panicky, she would have been a likely candidate for trouble. Jumping into the dinghy without oars, dropping the dinghy over the side without having the painter made fast . . . In the dark there are many possibilities, and grabbing, lunging, lurching or leaping to try and put things right might have been the moment when she herself went in.

Far-fetched? Not at all; that sort of thing happens time and again. I have a cutting by me from the journal of the Royal National Lifeboat Institution reporting an occasion when they sent out one of their Inshore Rescue Boats at Mudeford in Hampshire. 'A man had slipped and fallen overboard from the motor launch *Willynilly* when trying to weigh anchor. He had managed to hold on to the anchor chain, but his wife had gone to help him and she too had fallen overboard. The man had managed to climb back on board but his wife was swept away and was unable to regain the boat . . .'

Swept away – the tides run very strongly at Mudeford which is at the entrance to Christchurch Harbour, but happily the IRB's crew managed to rescue the lady, and all was well.

THE DANGERS OF GOING AFLOAT

Any sensible person who takes up boating recognises that it is a pastime which has its dangers, and tries to prepare himself against those dangers *as far as he can foresee them*. The difficult part of the task is the foreseeing. In this book I want to try and help that process, to stimulate the imagination, by presenting some experiences of trouble, and some ideas for either keeping out of it, or for coping with it if it cannot be avoided. What I write is based on experience, not my own of course, because nobody could suffer so many disasters and still be here to tell the tale, but experiences reported by the RNLI, and Coastguard, or other reputable sources. By seeing what has happened to others we should be able to make a reasoned, objective estimate of the risks of going afloat, and so be better prepared to deal with them.

It is possible to protect oneself to a large extent by some simple positive rules and practices, some of them so simple as to seem obvious. That chap who slipped quietly overboard late at night would probably agree that the *first* rule for anyone who goes boating is *don't fall overboard*.

At sea in blowy weather that particular skipper was in the habit of wearing a safety harness. Taking the dinghy ashore on a choppy night he would wear his excellent waterproof jacket with the built-in buoyancy. A prudent man. But what had never occurred to him before was that there's no difference between falling off a moored boat in a stream of 4 knots and falling off a boat which is sailing at 4 knots. Nor had it occurred to me until that night, though it is perfectly obvious. I wonder if it has ever crossed the minds of the many middle-aged men who are obliged to get out of their warm berths in the small hours by the pressing call of nature. Rather than disturb the whole ship with the clank and gurgle of the equipment provided, many of us prefer to stand on the deck's edge and admire the phosphorescence stimulated by our own personal contributions to the mighty ocean's flood.

Half-awake, a man perched on the edge of the deck may be in almost as much danger as one who should try the same antic on the window-ledge of a skyscraper. But we don't normally see the risk in those terms because we see the water as a playground, and are equally accustomed to the idea that falling in the water is a basic ingredient of comedy. On a fine day, in the right circumstances, an unexpected tumble into the water makes a good laugh. Yet . . .

Yet on the one occasion when a member of my crew has had to have hospital treatment as a result of a boating accident the incident itself was pure comedy. We capsized an overloaded dinghy in water so shallow that her keel was already touching the bottom. Indeed she would not have capsized if she had not been touching, for that was the reason for my asking one member of the party to step out and lighten our load. As he stepped he stumbled and fell – over went the boat, up into the air flew an oar, and there we were sitting in 3 inches of water, splattered with mud, and laughing ourselves silly, until we saw blood streaming down my wife's face. When that flying oar came down it had put a gash in her head that required several stitches.

Nobody could have seen the extraordinary behaviour of an oar in those particular circumstances, so you might say that this is a profitless story since nobody could prepare against such an accident. But it shows two things, first that small troubles can lead to bigger ones, and second that it is *always* folly to overload a dinghy in any circumstances – even in 3 inches of water. If I had shown more prudence and caution in the first place the business with the oar would not have happened.

And on a cruising boat, away from the services of the land, it is even more important to avoid or prevent accidents. Ashore, we are used to the idea that medical aid is always within reach, but on the sea you are on your own. If anything goes wrong with either ship or crew, then you have to be prepared to deal with it yourself – hence the need for the closest attention to every possible source of trouble.

I suppose it is true for life in general that small accidents are the first steps towards bigger ones. It is certainly true of boats, as anyone will know after he has had a few years of experience. For that reason even minor troubles must be eliminated as far as possible. As the editor of a yachting magazine I find that many people come new to boating with an inherent respect for the hazards of the water, but without any clear picture of what those hazards really are.

Let me illustrate again with another true story. The owner of an 18-foot, outboard-powered cabin boat took a party of friends for a fishing trip off the Yorkshire coast. It was a warm sunny day, with a blue sky and a calm sea, and they had no intention of going more than a mile offshore. All very straightforward, but that night they were picked up by the lifeboat after an air search had found them, in the last of the daylight. They were far off land and in a sea so rough that they would probably not have lasted through the night.

This narrow but happy escape came about because the skipper had not appreciated that a fresh westerly wind was blowing. The beach from which he launched the boat was backed by high cliffs which sheltered it and kept the water calm. Indeed it was still fairly calm when his engine came to a stop about a mile off the shore. At first there was no alarm. The two men started trying to put it right, but it was an unsuccessful effort that dragged on and on, and all the time they were working their boat was being blown farther out to sea, slowly at first, but faster as she came out from the land and into the stronger breeze.

As the day wore on and the boat drifted into an increasingly rough sea, dollops of cold spray came aboard, and the party began to feel the lack of warm and waterproof clothing. Nobody had thought of such things on that warm and sunny beach when they set out for a little pleasure jaunt. Nor had the skipper thought to drop anchor as soon as the engine stopped.

(Or perhaps he had no anchor, or an insufficient length of cable.) Nor had he thought to equip his little ship with red flares or orange smoke canisters, which would certainly have brought help if they had been used while the boat was still easily visible from the shore.

Lack of foresight, and a failure to appreciate that out there he would be on his own . . . yes, but he had taken one sensible precaution. He had left a note under the windscreen-wiper of his car, simply giving the name of his boat, the time of launching and the time expected to be back. A patrolling policeman was interested in a solitary car and trailer still in the car park at dusk. He saw the note, alerted the Coastguard, and so began the full-scale process of search and rescue.

KNOWING THE WORST

Although an engine failure, such as that recounted above, is a very common cause of a lifeboat sortie, such failures very rarely lead to loss of life. That fact I now know, though it was quite unknown to me just a few years ago when I sat down to write the first edition of this book. At that time there was no source of information, no record analysing the causes and nature of boating accidents. But in recent years the Royal National Lifeboat Institution has put its unrivalled and extensive records on computer tape, and that makes it possible to analyse and tabulate the essential facts contained in coxswains' reports of thousands of rescue missions.

As soon as I heard that this information had been recorded in a form that a computer could read, I asked the Institution (in my capacity as editor of *Boat Owner* magazine) if they would make special analyses of their records to see if private boat owners could learn where the most likely risks of boating lay. Although busy with analytical work of a different kind, directed towards their own operational needs, the Institution's staff responded willingly. Thus, for the first time we had available a factual guide to the real risks of boating and yachting.

A most important fact emerged at once. More than half of all boating fatalities were due to capsize. Death itself may have arisen from drowning or exposure, but the real cause was that the victim had been immersed in water by a capsize. Capsize also leads to a significant number of injuries, and it is quite clearly the most serious danger faced by those who go afloat.

A few, and quite a significant few, find themselves in the water as a consequence of falling overboard. But over a period of years the figures show quite clearly that capsize is the dominant type of accident that leads to death in boating. In fact, one can say that deaths from capsize equal or exceed those from all other categories of incidents – leaks, fire, swamping, man overboard, stranding and so forth.

The picture is confirmed by the records of the United States Coast Guard who find that capsize is the prime cause of deaths in pleasure boating in their country too.

What it boils down to is this: in every 100 pleasure boating fatalities you might save half a dozen if you could eliminate *all* accidental fires. You could eliminate a similar handful if you could obviate *all* leaks or swampings. You could eliminate four or five deaths if boats were never caught out in storms. Each of those would be worthwhile savings, and each is worth attention. But if you could do away with capsizes you would save between 50 and 60 of those 100 lives.

Evidently capsize is the type of incident most to be feared, so let us give some thought to it.

We can start on the basis that boats with cabins hardly ever capsize. This type of accident concerns small open craft, a fact which is confirmed by the RNLI's own analysis of their services. More than 90 per cent of fatal capsize incidents occur in open sailing dinghies, canoes, rowing boats, and open boats powered by outboard motors.

Like many other simple truths, this comes as no surprise when it is pointed out. Many small open rowing boats are used by sea anglers, chaps who are more concerned with catching fish than with seamanship or boathandling. Their boats are often loaded with more gear and people than they should properly carry, and with too little leg room it is all too easy for someone to stumble and throw his weight awkwardly on one side of the boat at just the wrong moment . . .

And a little boat like this is particularly vulnerable when the wind gets up and the sea becomes choppy. It is not that great waves immediately fill the boat with water. No, the sea gets her prey more subtly than that. Even quite small amounts of spray accumulating in the bottom of an open boat can add up to a significant weight – and a freely-moving weight at that. With the slightest inclination of the boat, that weight of water runs to the low side and makes matters immediately worse. And in an overcrowded boat, with booted feet, boxes of bait, rods, crates of beer and the like, even an attempt to bail can result in a disturbance of bodies which may upset a small boat.

With sailing dinghies capsize occurs in a different way. Except in the lightest breeze the sails themselves exert a powerful capsizing force on the boat – a force which is counter-balanced by the body weight of an agile crew. The more sail you carry the faster you go – and the greater the capsizing tendency and the greater balancing demand on the crew. Quite rightly, people are taught how to right a capsized dinghy. Quite wrongly, the idea is put about that so long as you know how to right your boat it does not matter how often you let her capsize. Sadly, it *does* matter to those few who each year find themselves unable, just this once, to right their capsized dinghies. (On page 125 you will find an account of a true, and typical, incident which illustrates my point.)

Regrettably, capsizing is now so commonplace in dinghy racing that many dinghy sailors seem to feel that to turn your boat over is perfectly normal, and that keeping her the right way up is old-maidish and cissy. But it should be quite obvious that no true seaman would allow his boat to be turned over if he could avoid it. While it *may* be safe to capsize your dinghy in a race, with a club safety boat in attendance, it is a very foolhardy thing to do when you are at sea on your own. Self-reliance is the essence of seamanship.

I have talked about capsize because it is the dominant cause of death in boating accidents. It is also one of the two main reasons for lifeboat calls. Between them, capsize and engine failure account for more than half of all lifeboat launches, but although engine failure keeps the lifeboatmen busy, it results in virtually no fatalities.

With so much concentration upon fatal boating accidents I feel that I may be spreading a certain amount of gloom. I hope not, because boating is in fact a very safe pastime. In recent years the number of people drowned in pleasure boating accidents in Britain has been around the 100 mark – only about 15 per cent of drownings from all causes. That total is well below the number drowned in swimming, and well below the number of small children who drown annually because they are allowed to play near water.

In short, we can claim that boating, in which very large numbers of people participate, is a very safe pastime. And having established that, we can then do our best to make it even safer.

1. Bumps, Bruises ... and
Even Broken Ribs

Bruises seem to be an almost inevitable result of even one weekend aboard a boat, and women seem to be the worst sufferers. No doubt they bruise more easily than the complementary sex, and they tend to be shorter in the leg – a fact which is of significance when it comes to getting up from the cabin to the cockpit, or from the cockpit to the deck.

In fact many minor (and some major) accidents come simply from the ups and downs and awkward corners on board a boat, and to some extent designers and builders are to blame. A day at the Boat Show will always yield its crop of boats with traps and pitfalls – but often these matters can be put right by the owner himself, and if that is possible, then an awkward companionway need not be a deterrent to buying an otherwise satisfactory boat.

HANDHOLDS

Because a boat heels, and rolls, and pitches, more care is needed in designing for human movement than in a fixed building. In fact wherever people may go in a boat there should be a firm foothold and a good handhold. If you can find those two attributes in a boat then you know that she has been designed (or built) by someone whose experience extends beyond the drawing board, and reaches out to sea. With the boat lurching about it can be a risky business simply moving from one end of the cabin to the other. A heavy sea will hurtle a man right across a cabin and when he picks himself up he may find that he has a broken nose, a broken arm or a broken rib.

The answer is some kind of handhold – usually a rail along the underside of the deckhead, so that you cannot find yourself in the centre of the cabin and out of reach of either bulkhead or either side of the ship. Some boats have vertical posts (like the buses) – we have them on our own boat as a matter of fact, where they also serve another purpose. A good handhold is very welcome in the w.c. compartment too, where it is perhaps of slightly more value to the men but nevertheless of value to all. I know one burly fellow who, while standing in such a compartment, adopted the usual trick of bracing himself by thrusting his elbows against the bulkheads on either side. She was a fibreglass boat, and the bulkheads were too flexible to give a good grip. The ship lurched and my friend went backwards through the rather flimsy plywood door, on across the ship and through the door of the hanging locker on the opposite side. At that stage he was sincerely hoping that the hull side was somewhat more stoutly built . . . Happily it was, or the hanging clothes absorbed the shock. No harm done – except to those doors – but a stout handrail would have been very welcome.

To be able to brace oneself in the galley is obviously very important, and since it may be necessary to use both hands, the well-equipped ship has a broad webbing strap passing round the cook's hips, against which she can brace herself with her feet. In this department there is a real danger of scalding, so if there is to be cooking while the boat is under way the cook would be wise to wear oilskins at her (or his) work.

The step or steps which lead from cabin to cockpit are often an obvious source of trouble because they are awkwardly positioned, too small, slippery when wet, not visible when stepping down from the cockpit, or too near some sharp locker corner or the like. One of the most common faults, which I find in brand-new boats year after year is that one has to make too big a step. Sometimes the distance is enough to tax the legs of an average man, let alone a tiny boatwife. And if in addition to making the steps themselves both difficult and dangerous, the designer has failed to provide handholds, then obviously he is no seaman. (One begins to be suspicious about the rest of his work if one finds such an omission.)

Good handholds are sometimes not to be found when making that other important transition – from cockpit to deck. They are probably more to be desired when coming down than when going up, but it is folly to be without them. Especially so because on deck there are other hazards – sheet winches, cleats, eyebolts and other fittings which can trip you up. Broken toes are a not uncommon 'yachtsman's injury', sometimes embellished by a wetting if the victim trips so badly that he goes overboard too.

FOOTWORK

It is difficult to keep a boat's deck clear of all such obstructions, especially if she is a sailing boat, but it is worth trying. Sometimes a look around will reveal ways in which improvement can be made: sometimes one is driven to it by sheer exasperation. But on the whole it must surely be better to try and take corrective action before you have trouble.

A very common cause of danger on deck is the loose rope – not because it catches around the ankles, but because it rolls beneath the foot if you tread on it. Worse than any banana-skin. And so is a Terylene sail – *surprisingly* slippery. The prudent skipper tries to arrange his boat so that such hazards are rare, but he also teaches his crew to step round them when they do exist.

Decks themselves should have a non-slip surface. Sometimes boats which are moulded in resin and glass have large glossy areas with small non-slip patches at certain points where one is supposed to stand and work. These treated spaces may be on the foredeck where one stands to bring up the anchor, or around the mast where halyard work and reefing are done. In my view that is not a satisfactory scheme. In the first place you have to get to and from these specially prepared standing points. Secondly, it is just not possible to say where you may or may not have to stand at some time or other. And it is in times of trouble – in a rough sea with a broken boom perhaps – that you may find yourself having to stand and work at an unusual point on deck; that's a fine time to wish you were on a non-slip surface! The only safe rule, as I see it, is to have a good non-slip finish *wherever* you may possibly want to get a foot-hold. (And one should not forget the business of climbing aboard from the dinghy.)

Precisely what sort of finish is best for non-slip properties is hard to define. Many people swear by the good old laid deck of bare teak, but not many of us have that sort of boat. Wooden decks of ply can be made thoroughly skid-proof by coating with sand-paint, either obtained ready-mixed from the chandler's shop or made up at home. (One owner I know paints his deck with Sandtex, an exterior finish for houses, and says that it gives excellent results.)

A similar paint can be used on the decks of moulded resin-glass boats, not forgetting that a special primer may be needed to get a good key the first time it is applied. All such paints have the disadvantage that the better they are for grip the harsher they are on clothes and skin. Non-slip paint will easily wear through a pair of trousers in half a summer if you have the sort of boat where the helmsman habitually sits on the sidedeck.

Some wooden decks are coated with Trakmark, which is a PVC-surfaced material embossed with a fine diamond or pinhead pattern. This is moderately non-slip, but not so good in my experience as the emery-cloth effect of sand-paint.

A Trakmark pattern is permanently moulded into the decks of some resin-glass boats. On the whole I doubt the efficacy of a moulded pattern though it must evidently be better than nothing at all. There is difficulty in getting sharp edges to the pattern – the nature of the material tends towards rounded corners. And even if the edges are pretty sharp when the boat is new they round off with time and wear. Although I have found some boats which had a very effective moulded-in deck pattern when new I would still prefer a good scratchy paint.

A very useful proprietary material called Safety-Walk is made by the Three-Ms company. This is like strips of emery-cloth, about one inch wide with an adhesive backing. Although one naturally suspects that the adhesive will lose its grip after a few months of rain and sunshine, the contrary seems to be true. I have used strips of this stuff on a varnished bowsprit, and even after six years it showed no inclination to come unstuck. And it really is non-slip – rather useful for points where one has to step down to the cockpit or the cabin.

These minor hazards on a small boat are commonly made very much more dangerous by hasty movements. A headsail sheet gets foul of a cleat at the foot of the mast when the boat is tacking, and some well-meaning member of the party leaps into action – only to finish up with a black eye or a stubbed toe or occasionally something worse. One has to cultivate the art of moving sedately but swiftly, taking everything in good time and acting in the mood of the time-honoured saying 'one hand for the ship and one hand for yourself'. Dashing about on a small boat invariably leads to injury sooner or later, and with something so 'knobbly' as a boat any fall can have quite bad consequences. There are three specially bad falling areas into an open forehatch, into the cockpit, and overboard. Everyone should make it a rigid principle of his life's philosophy *never to fall overboard*, and it would be a good idea to say the same of falls into cockpits and down hatches. I have tried both kinds, on several occasions, so I do know what I'm talking about!

ROPEWORK, AND MIND YOUR HANDS

A common cause of serious falls on boats is the breaking rope. The victim may be swigging on the main halyard, when suddenly it breaks and back he goes. *Where* he goes will depend on the amount of forethought he has given to the chance of such an event. If he has given it no thought at all he may go straight overboard, or, worse, he may injure his spine by falling back on to a vast steel anchor windlass. The wiser, more experienced, or better-taught hand, will position himself where the least damage seems likely to result. Usually that means lining one's back up with the shrouds which act as a safety net – of sorts.

Any rope on which one is hauling may come home suddenly, whether because it breaks, a hitch slips or for any other reason. The tug-o'-war team that collapses backwards on the grass makes good film comedy, and no harm done. In a boat it is a matter to be taken seriously because one is not falling back on grass – just take a look behind you next time you are heaving on a warp or breaking the anchor out.

A most fearful practice that one grieves to see done all too frequently is to take a turn of a rope around the hand in order to get a better grip. It is a practice which is not necessarily *always* dangerous, but the only way to be sure of avoiding those times when it will be dangerous is to make a rule *never* to do it. In fact, of course, it is a thing one tends to do when the load is hardest to hold, and that is the very time when the risk is greatest.

If one has a turn of rope around either hand or wrist there may come a moment when it is impossible to free it. Yet the only truly important point is that one must always be free to let go whenever it is necessary. We have all of us giggled a little over the sight of some poor woman (it usually falls to the put-upon

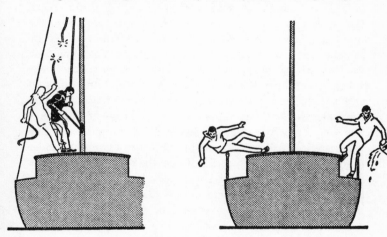

A breaking rope has been the cause of many a fall, and (like an actor) the wise sailorman tries to fall softly if he must. The chap swigging on the halyard (*left*) takes up a position where he will fall against the shrouds if the rope breaks. The sketch on the right is a reminder that although most modern boats have guard-rails, a man on a coachroof may easily be pitched right over them. If properly made, the rail should be amply strong enough to support his weight, even if leaning out from the side deck (*right*).

wives, I notice) hanging on to a mooring buoy until it seems that her arm is about to be wrenched off. So long as she *can* let go, well and good, but I know one fellow who lost two fingers because he took a turn round his hand. The boat was not a very big one – no more than a 5-tonner – but the combined effect of wind and tide dragged his hand against the sharp-edged cheek plate of the stemhead fitting and he just could not free himself.

It is very easy for a writer to lay down the law and point out the risks, but it is surprising how long a time may pass before one finds a constructive answer. I am ashamed to recall how long it took before I adopted the simple solution to the problem of a wife whose strength was too often overtaxed by the effort needed to bring the mooring home. For some time we had carried on board one of those automatic snaphooks which have a line attached and slip off the end of a boatstaff with a quite gentle pull. We kept it in a locker – waiting for that day when we should come alongside some imagined quay, or a pile with a mooring ring, and it was not until one windy day when my wife had twice hooked the buoy and twice had to let it go again (very sensibly) that I saw the simple and obvious answer. From that day forward we used that gadget, and with the line made fast to the samson post all she has to do is to get the hook on the strop of the buoy, or on the mooring chain itself. From that moment boat and mooring are linked, and it is up to me to bring the chain home at leisure.

I feel that some apology should be offered for putting forward something so simple and obvious, something that so many other people must have done before me. But observation suggests that I am not the only one who sometimes puts himself and his family to unnecessary and risky muscular strain simply because I have not made the effort to think out a better technique. So I offer this tale as an example that a little brain, (yes *very* little!) can take the place of a great deal of brawn.

Hands suffer a good deal in boating. If anything has to be done it is our hands which lead the action – they go to steady us along the deck and perhaps grab a frayed wire, or a badly-finished splice with nasty little ends sticking out. They go to fend off another boat or a quayside – or they may do if their owner has not trained himself to regulate his reflexes with a little thought. Though one may put out hand or foot to separate a couple of dinghies, it is a practice not to be risked with cabin boats. One can never be sure quite what will happen, just how the boats will meet or what forces will be generated. If a fender cannot be interposed then one must look intelligently for some spot where hand or foot can be brought to bear without risk of injury. If an approaching craft is a sailing boat then her shrouds are likely to be the best if you can reach them, because they flex and because they cannot trap you. Lifelines and guardrails are another choice, but a foot or a hand between two sizeable boats, or between boat and quay – *never*.

Likewise, a rope should not be allowed to run through the hand. For one thing it blisters and burns. For another there may be a bight or loop in the rope which will catch hand or finger.

There is one minor accident which children too commonly suffer to their hands, and that is to have them pinched between dinghy and boat. What a rotten start to a nice weekend on the water! The family pile into the dinghy and off they go under oars or outboard towards their boat. Father brings the dinghy alongside a little too fiercely, all unaware that little Linda has her fingers curled over the gunwale. What ensues is best glossed over, and one only hopes that it is not as bad as it sounds.

In fact children are usually safer against tumbles and

bruises than adults, partly because the boat is relatively bigger for them, partly because they have a lower centre of gravity, and partly because they are more resilient. But they do need special thought. Young skins and young eyes are very susceptible to the intensified sunlight that is found on the water. A child in a dinghy can easily lose an oar and tumble in trying to retrieve it. Some sharp corners which are at thigh-height for an adult may be at eye-height for a child.

Long hair, and anoraks with draw strings at the neck may make unexpected dangers for children and adults alike. They are things that would not be permitted in a factory, yet one wonders how many people think of an outboard motor with whirling flywheel, or an inboard engine with its casing removed, as an open and unguarded machine? Yet such they are, and if you have seen a woman trailing her long hair over the belt-drive to the alternator of a 30 h.p. diesel, you won't need any urging from me. If it were not for the fact that we don't want too much grue I could tell a true story concerning a man and an outboard starting cord whose knotted end jammed in the flywheel of the motor . . . but let's leave it to the imagination. Engines are not the only wild beasts on a boat – a flogging sail can do fearful damage, and it should be approached warily, getting control of it by the sheet if possible.

I am not trying to say that these are *the* dangers. They are examples of many in boats which have no direct connection with the sea. One may have lifejackets, distress flares, and all the rest, and then lose an eye to one of those rubber cords which have wicked hooks on the end. It is not possible to foresee everything, but a rather pessimistic imagination can be a help!

2. Don't Fall Overboard ...
but If You Do

There are plenty of ways of falling overboard. One friend of mine went over from a river boat as he brought her into a lock; trying to hang on and bridge the ever-widening gap between boat and lock-side he finally over-reached himself and tumbled quietly in. The lock-keeper retrieved him with a boathook, brought him to the stone steps, and then brought the boat back alongside with the boathook so that the victim could step aboard. Dripping wet he stepped down into the cabin where his wife, occupied with the preparation of lunch, said simply, 'I didn't know it was raining dear, you really must get your waterproofs on.' (Yes, it's perfectly true.)

That is a classical way of falling in, of course, and it usually attracts more attention. It can also have a less happy outcome when the boat is in a lock or against a stone harbour wall, especially if anyone slips *between* the vessel and the wall.

It is possible to fall overboard unobserved even when other people are on deck. There was the case of an owner who was 'assisted' over the bows of a small sailing cruiser by the genoa jib which he was attempting to muzzle. As he surfaced he was close by the stern of the boat, where he managed to grab the rudder which made a convenient step. A few seconds later he was tapping the shoulder of a surprised helmsman who believed him still to be on the foredeck in the flurry of canvas.

Apart from the fact that both men in the above incidents went over unnoticed, these stories illustrate the two aspects of the matter – first, going over (which is very easy) and second, getting back (which is usually very hard).

GUARDRAILS, LIFELINES

Prevention is better than cure of course, and in that respect modern boats and modern crews are far better prepared than they were a couple of generations ago. Even the smallest cabin boat nowadays has some sort of rail round the deck, and even if not fitted all round, it will be found at certain important points. The contrast with boats of the period before the Second World War is quite remarkable. Though some of the larger vessels of those days did have rails around their decks, the majority of craft up to about 30 feet in length had no protection. And even the few big yachts which did have rails were usually without the bowrail, which has since come to be called the pulpit for obvious reasons. I am sure that had anyone fitted a pulpit to a 5-tonner in those days he would have been an object of ridicule, not on any practical grounds but simply because it would have been thought to *look* wrong.

Nobody says *that* now, even if there may still be some people who object to the term 'pushpit' for the after rail which can be so valuable at sea. (In passing, I would be very happy to put up a strong defence of that useful word, despite its punning origin, just as I am eager to help the introduction of a new noun into our language for any new thing that needs a label. If one has to write about things then one soon learns the limitations of a static and crystallised vocabulary, and in this case there *is* a need for a word to define that form of rail which is not the same as the older, stouter and more ornate taffrail. But let that be – those who don't wish to say 'pushpit' out loud need not do so, but when the word falls on their delicate ears I am sure it will be meaningful.)

It is fair to say that there is now general agreement that, except for open boats and certain half-decked racing classes, all boats should be fitted with some sort of fence around the deck. The three most important considerations in its design are that it should be strong enough, that it should be high enough, so that one cannot easily fall over it, and finally, one should not be able to fall under or through it.

A height of 2 feet is the generally accepted minimum for the guardrail around the boat, which is commonly of wire stretched tightly around a set of tubular stanchions. Whether the stanchions are made of stainless steel or of galvanised mild steel, the crucial point is the attachment to the deck. There are many types of fitting on the market, and some do not inspire my confidence. One has to remember that the purpose of the fitting is to take the shock of a man falling against the top end of a stanchion, or on to the wire at some point between stanchions. With a leverage of 2 feet, that can exert a very high load at the base which must therefore be designed so that well-spaced bolts can secure it to the deck. And if the base is strong the deck itself can easily be overloaded, so one must be sure that the load goes either into a deckbeam or that it is well spread by some kind of reinforcement. In practice most modern boats are provided with proper reinforcement in way of the stanchion bases, but there are always exceptions. When one is inspecting a new boat with a view to purchase it is entirely fair and reasonable to *try* to break the stanchions away by leaning or lurching against them. If you care to go so far as to *throw* yourself against a guardrail or pulpit, so much the better. If it should break then the builder has no cause for complaint about your boisterous behaviour for you will have done him (as well as yourself) a good service in revealing a dangerous weakness.

31

Should you want to approach the matter more scientifically, each stanchion alone should be able to withstand a horizontal force of 150 lb, applied at the top.

With the ordinary 2-foot high (60 cm) guardwire there is normally a second wire at half height so that one cannot fall *through*. These wires often pass through drillings in the stanchions, where they must be protected against chafe. A short length of copper tube is fitted in each hole for that purpose, and has its ends belled out both to provide a fair run for the wire and to keep it in place.

The natural shape of a boat means that the guardwire runs in a fore-and-aft curve, making a very effective shape for any outward load, so long as the ends of the wire are well secured. In other words, a wire can take the load only in tension, and when checking the fitness of one's own vessel that point must be remembered. In bigger craft, where weight is not so important, there is much to be said for having a guardrail of steel tube, or even of timber. Very effective safety rails can be made from the galvanised tube known as 'water barrel' which is inexpensive, can be bought from any builders' merchant, and provides stiffness as well as tensile strength.

Sometimes the area of the cockpit is omitted from the protection of the guardrail and, in my view, that is a mistake. The motion of a small boat at sea can be surprisingly lively and it is quite easy for a member of the crew to be pitched over the lee side or to tumble backwards over the weather side. Indeed, as a general rule it is wise to assume that a boat will have guardrails all round unless there is some very good reason to the contrary. And although the current convention stipulates a height of 2 feet there is no reason why one should not go higher provided that the base fitments can be made sufficiently strong to cope with the extra leverage that may be exerted.

32

In some boats, especially the smaller ones, the rail is lower than 2 feet. In such cases there is the obvious drawback that a low rail may serve as little better than a trip wire nicely judged to catch you behind the knees and help you overboard. Yet where boom clearance or some other factor imposes a restriction an owner may quite sensibly adopt a lower rail so long as he recognises that he had better crawl forward when necessary, rather than try to proceed in a dignified but dangerous upright attitude. In this connection it is worth recording that the Royal Ocean Racing Club specifies a height of 24 inches for competitors, and that the smaller boats of the Junior Offshore Group are permitted a lower height.

It does not do to be dogmatic about these things. Many small yachts have been successfully sailed round the world and on other long oceanic passages without benefit of any type of guardrail around their decks ... nevertheless I cannot see much advantage in *not* having them.

Even though one's boat is fitted with strong guardrails at a sensible height, it will still be necessary to hold on when going forward in heavy weather and proper handrails should be fitted. Where handrails are not possible then one must devise a way of getting about the deck so that there is always something to hang on to. Furthermore most people now wear a safety harness which fits around the chest and over the shoulders (like the harness used to restrain an infant in its pram), with a length of line with a springhook which can be clipped to the guardrail, the shrouds or any other convenient point.

If properly designed, such a harness will drag a person through the water in a controlled attitude and without putting any undue strain on his back. A harness attached low down, near the waist and running round the small of the back may well do harm when the wearer is brought up with a jerk. Of course, it is a nuisance to put the harness on, especially if you are already cluttered up with warm clothes, oilskins and perhaps some kind of buoyancy gear too. Nevertheless, it is wise to accustom oneself to wearing harness whenever the weather is bad, and *always* at night. It is also very sensible to wear it when sailing alone, and not only in heavy weather. The fate of the single-hander who slips overboard, even for the most trivial or laughable reason, is an unenviable one, especially since he is tempted to lash the tiller and leave the boat to herself if there is some little job to be done on deck. And nowadays self-steering devices are quite common. So for one reason or the other one cannot rely on the idea that if the helm is let fly the boat will round up of her own accord and come to a standstill. Perhaps it would be wise to heave to, but people do *like* to keep going.

When sailing alone I rather like to have the dinghy astern on an unusually long painter, though a long and buoyant warp might do as well for a sufficiently agile person. The advantage of the dinghy over the warp is that it is easier to board the dinghy first, especially if she is an inflatable. If, on the other hand, it is to be a matter of a climb up high topsides from the water, then a ropeladder should be so arranged that it can easily be pulled over the side from the water.

The real answer is to wear harness, and that applies whether one is sailing alone or not. Then all you have to do is to make it a rule that the harness is always attached to the boat. I know one experienced and competent helmswoman who was washed out of her cockpit while wearing *unattached* harness – and she did know perfectly well that she was approaching dangerously rough water ... The originator of the personal harness as a normal piece of yacht's chandlery was Peter Haward, and he also established the technique of having two snaphooks on the line, one at the full length and the other about half-way. Apart from the fact that this allows you to use a shortened line, it also makes it possible to clip one hook to a secure point before you unclip the other. But that step-by-step progress is rather tedious, and a more practical solution is to arrange a line from the cockpit to the foredeck to which the snaphook can be clipped. Just how this jackstay can be rigged must depend on the boat herself – sometimes one can rig a pair of them, one to port and the other to starboard. Or it may even be possible to rig a single continuous line which starts at the cockpit, goes forward round the mast, and comes back to the cockpit again. In that case it may be possible to get to all parts of the ship without unclipping the harness-line.

Sometimes the boatbuilder himself provides the attachment for your harness-line, thus showing himself to be one of those who take their responsibilities seriously. But whether you have a provision or not, the aim should be to use the harness in such a way that it prevents you from falling overboard. It's far better to stay on the ship, even though Peter Haward has demonstrated that with his harness you can fall in at 9 knots and be towed along without harm.

In practice, the preventive use of the harness may mean that techniques will have to be thought out carefully. If, for example, you have to go to the mast to reef the mainsail, you may find it best to work on the lee side of the ship, with the harness attached to the weather shrouds. Some people like this position of hanging back, as it were and looking uphill. On the other hand such a scheme may not fit in with the position of the shrouds and the reefing gear on your particular boat. In any case, I think that most people feel happier on the 'uphill' side. Much depends on the proportions of the boat: it may prove more practical to have a single jackstay running along the centre line of the coachroof, from cockpit to mast. That can sometimes work very well, for with a harness-line made up to the right length it can be quite impossible for you to go overboard from either side of the ship. In such a scheme a similar jackstay may be needed forward of the mast, though it is sometimes possible to run a single line from the cockpit, close by the foot of the mast to terminate 2 or 3 feet further forward. Another method is to use mast-track, screwed and bolted to the deck. In that case there has to be a slide with an eye to which the harness-line is clipped, and it is necessary to have the slide at 'your end' of the track when you want to clip on.

In my view it is highly desirable for the single-hander to try and arrange the jackstay so that he is clipped on while at the helm. (And in this context a single-hander should include the solitary helmsman on deck while other members of a small crew are sleeping below.) If the jackstay runs right aft, then the helmsman can move forward without having to remember to clip on. Furthermore, he is protected while actually at the helm: in many small craft it is possible to be pitched out of the cockpit in heavy weather – even when not overcome by drowsiness.

It is pretty obvious that a jackstay, or another attachment for a safety line must be strongly fitted, preferably with through-bolts or something equally reliable.

The business of putting the harness on over heavy clothing is something of a deterrent, and I believe that there is a great deal to be said for the type of waterproof jacket which embodies both harness and buoyancy. These garments are expensive, though there is not much in it if you compare the cost to the total of jacket, buoyancy waistcoat and harness bought separately. In British waters one probably *wants* to wear a waterproof jacket on those very occasions when it is wise to wear harness and buoyancy, whereas in warmer climates one might want to wear only the harness. (Though as a matter of fact few of the long-distance trade-wind sailors seem to have worn harness, in spite of the severe rolling that most small craft suffer on those ocean passages.)

Buoyancy gear forms the subject of another chapter, but there is one more point that should be made about harness. If you should go overboard wearing a harness that is not clipped to a boat it can still be of value, because it will provide a lifting point for those who are trying to get you back on board.

GETTING BACK ON BOARD

Getting back aboard a boat at sea, especially in water-logged clothing, can be extremely difficult – perhaps impossible – even for a fit man who is not yet weakened by exposure. Here again there is no simple or universal answer – all one can do is to point to some of the methods which have been successful, and also to some of the *ideas* which have been put forward even though they may never have been proved in a real emergency. It must then be up to each skipper to decide what will suit his boat and his family (or crew). Then, having worked out what seems a good technique the crew should be given practice in it. But I fear that practising man-overboard drill is something that most of us are going to do 'when we get round to it'. We are likely to be still waiting to get round to it when we finally have to do it in earnest.

One thing a good skipper might sensibly do is to go overboard while the boat is at her mooring, wearing full clothing, and see for himself the problems of re-boarding his own boat. Although that is not the same as going overboard while the boat is under way it does give good practice in the actual re-boarding process, even though it omits other parts of the real man-overboard situation.

The first thing that will become obvious is the gravity of the problem if no help is available from on board the boat herself, as would be the situation of the single-hander. This will at once suggest the idea of fitting some sort of foothold or step on the rudder or the transom – or both. Handholds will be needed, too, and one simple way of combining the two is to make a short rope ladder which is permanently attached to the boat and stowed on the after-deck in such a way that it can be brought into action without delay. The single-hander will have to devise a way of deploying such a ladder while he is still in the water, which almost certainly implies that there must be some sort of tripping line permanently dangling . . . The idea may not attract, but the aesthetic loss may prove a lifesaving gain at some time in the future.

A ropeladder is not an easy thing to use of course, so practice is indicated. Fixed steps will probably be better, if the shape of the boat makes them feasible, but even the most ingenious handyman will find them difficult to arrange on a boat with a counter stern. Likewise the rudder contributes nothing to this problem if it is not transom-hung.

Small, folding metal steps such as those supplied by Simpson Lawrence can be had from chandlers, and these may be the solution for some boats. They can also be useful in the ordinary process of boarding from the dinghy, especially for women. A patent system, called Mastep, which has links and steps moulded in plastics, might do very well. It is assembled link by link, to make any desired length. But fixed wooden steps may be equally practical and a good deal cheaper, and it is quite practicable to fit them in such a way that they are neither an eyesore nor an obstruction when coming alongside – at least not if you have a suitably shaped hull.

The really agile single-hander may even be satisfied with a bight of rope over the stern into which he can get his foot. Fair enough, but it must be accessible from the water and permanently made fast on deck. In my view, some such ropes should be permanently ready for action on any boat, even where there are other crew members available to give a hand. My own practice is to have a line available on each side of the boat which can be dropped down to the water without a moment's delay. *In theory*, both these lines are lowered whenever I am sailing single-handed: at other times they are lightly restrained at deck level, but ready to be dropped instantly if necessary. I adopted these lines only after a frightening incident had opened my eyes. Again it was my wife who was the victim. She went overboard at sea as a result of some rather unusual events which are not really pertinent. Having brought the boat about I came up to leeward of Dorothy who by this time was feeling somewhat waterlogged (heavy clothing, no buoyancy, no harness) and in need of help. I leaned over the side and took her hands in mine, giving her a chance to rest and to breathe freely with her head well clear of the water. Fine – but it was stalemate. On the deck, just a few feet away was a bathing ladder which would be the means by which she could get up to me or I could get down and help her. *But I did not dare to let go of her hands.*

Luckily, it was possible to reach the staysail sheet with one hand and pass a bight of it down to her. From that point forward it was a relatively simple matter to complete the job, but if that sheet had not been handy I should ultimately have been forced to leave hold of her hands, and that is a thing one is very loath to do in such circumstances.

In fact our boat has bumkins with chainstays running down to the waterline, so there was another handhold available to which I could have transferred her. But that is a rarity which most boats do not enjoy, so I think the message is pretty clear. It was certainly clear enough for me to rig those lifelines, *and* to organise a new stowage for the bathing ladder so that it would be more accessible.

I believe that a bathing ladder whose bottom rung extends at

39

least a foot below the water level, and preferably even deeper, is a *primary* piece of safety equipment. It is easily the best way to get a conscious man aboard, and it is also the best way for a helper to go over the side and secure a line to an unconscious or injured man.

Supposing that no such ladder is available, and that there is no ropeladder either, the simplest form of aid is a bight of rope for the foot. But unless the victim is agile and circumstances are ideal, it is wise to take the extra precaution of securing a line around his chest and under his armpits. A member of the crew can keep shortening in so as to keep this line short and to ensure that any ground made good is not lost. With such a line it is possible to use a step-by-step technique. First a bight of rope is lowered to a length which allows the man in the water to get his foot in it and 'step' up by about six inches. Then his bodyline is shortened in and made fast so that he cannot slip back, and then the foot rope is shortened so that he can raise himself another six inches by the power of his own leg muscles.

To make this procedure really effective the bodyline should lead from a high point, since one will ultimately want to have the man's shoulders above the gunwale level of the boat. Thus a halyard, or the topping lift, might be employed. It is a slow process, but it is one which I know has enabled a small woman to get a large man aboard. It relieved her of much of the muscular work.

Sometimes it may be easier for the victim to climb aboard a dinghy as an intermediate stage. It is not at all easy for most people to pull themselves in over the transom of a rigid dinghy, and although the help of another person in the boat may solve that problem most yacht's tenders are really too small to make that kind of thing a safe operation. There is too much risk that both chaps will finish up in the water. With an

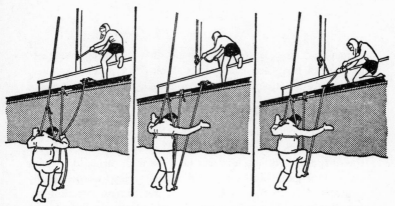

Getting a water-logged man back on to a boat can be almost impossible unless ingenuity is used. The method above has been used in earnest by at least one woman. Having secured a halyard to the man, she also provided a bight of rope for his foot. Man raised himself by own leg muscle to 'standing' position. Woman then shortened in on halyard to hold what had been gained, and followed by shortening foot rope so that man could take another step up. And so on step by step, using man's leg muscle and woman's brain. The drawing below shows a possible method, using a sheet winch. Best of all is a bathing ladder, but it is always worth trying and practising any idea that seems appropriate to the boat and her equipment.

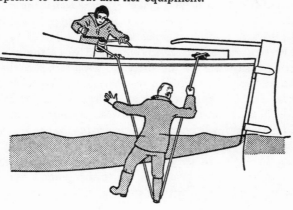

inflatable dinghy, on the other hand, it is a different story because these boats are usually very stable (except in the smallest
'beach-toy' sizes) and their soft, rounded shape makes it easier
to get aboard. So if an inflatable is being towed astern it may
well prove most effective for a crew member to get aboard it
and retrieve his man from there. Even if the inflatable is
stowed on deck it could be well worth launching her specially for
the purpose. (Though all must be done with care and without
haste. One can easily see that a too-hasty leap into a dinghy
could lead to further troubles. 'I'll get him in the dinghy,'
says our hero, leaping in and casting off, only to find that he has
no oars . . .)

Another procedure which I have seen recommended, though
I have no experience of it, makes use of the gangplank that is
carried aboard some large boats, especially those which berth
in marinas or Mediterranean-style harbours. It involves rigging
the plank alongside the boat, lying fore and aft, so that its
lower end dips beneath the water. It thus forms a miniature
slip, or a walkway similar to those which kindly people provide
to help ducks come ashore from a pond. If it can be rigged it
would obviously be helpful to a man in the water, but it is one
of those things in which all the crew must be practised if it is
to be brought into action when wanted.

The problem is very much simplified when the victim is
wearing a harness, even though it was not attached to the boat
when he went overboard. In that case one has a ready-made
means of attachment. In boats which have halyard winches it
would be no great problem to lift even an unconscious man
from the water if a halyard can be secured to his harness. Or, in
boats so equipped, the fall from a davit can be used.

Another merit of the harness is that one may be able to
latch on to it with a boathook. Up to this point I have been
concerned only with the problem of getting the chap back on

board after you have made contact with him. But even a good helmsman may not always be able to bring the vessel within arm's reach of the person in the water, and it may therefore be necessary to bridge the gap either by throwing a line, or by reaching out with a boathook. The boathook is in itself a dangerous instrument (though a bruise or two is better than drowning) but it has the advantage that it can be better aimed than a thrown rope. Moreover it can be effective if the victim is helpless. A useful form of boathook in either case is the kind fitted with a patent snaphook which has a line attached and comes free of the shaft. This makes it possible to *pass* a line, rather than to throw it, while if the victim is helpless it may be possible to snap the hook to his harness or (a remote chance) his clothing.

The permutations and possibilities in this problem of getting somebody back on board are virtually endless, depending on the boat, the people, the weather and other circumstances. But in my view three things stand out. First there is the need for places where the victim can get a handhold. Second there is the need to get a line made fast around him if there is going to be any delay at all in getting him in – in other words if he cannot just clamber back immediately. Third, that a good bathing ladder is one of the most valuable items of safety equipment to have on board.

But when it is a case of man overboard, getting him out of the water is only half the story. Before one can attempt that, the boat must be brought within reach of the man, and the manoeuvres to do that seem worthy of a chapter to themselves.

3. 'Man Overboard'

It may seem odd that I have had so much to say about getting a man (or woman) back on board before turning to the event that must precede it – bringing the boat to the man. It could be said that this is not the logical order, and it is certainly not the order in which things happen, but it was the order that came naturally to my mind. Perhaps it was because I was subconsciously funking the business of wagging a finger and admonishing all readers that the only good advice to give about 'man overboard' is to practise and practise again.

But there was also the reason that if one can suggest the great difficulty of getting back on board a cruising boat from the water, perhaps more people will take good care not to go overboard at all. It cannot be stressed too often that that is the most important safety precept of all.

As with all the matters we have been considering, there are many permutations depending on circumstances. If an infant should fall off a yacht with several others aboard it can be expected that one or more will immediately dive after it. That is one situation that could well arise in 'easy' circumstances, perhaps even on a day when people are already in bathing gear and are still barely dry from their last swim. In stark contrast is the situation in which one newly-wed young man found himself when he fell off the stern of the motor cruiser he had chartered

44

for his honeymoon. His new wife, innocent of all boating knowledge, was down in the cabin at that moment, but when she came back into the cockpit and saw her frantically-waving husband some hundreds of yards astern she quickly took charge of the steering wheel and turned back – a manoeuvre that brought him more terror than comfort when he saw that powerful craft bearing down on him at about 15 knots and thought of those twin, whirling propellers . . . In the event, his wife found and closed the throttles, and circling slowly round him was finally able to get the boat out of gear in accordance with his shouted instructions. He then swam to the boat and after more struggles managed to clamber aboard.

RETRACING YOUR STEPS

For our purposes we must try to picture not the rarer eventualities, but more typical incidents. Of these the first is the case where a crew member is discovered to be absent and therefore presumed overboard, even though nobody saw him go. At that point one can only hope that the boat has been sailing on a known compass course – which is always a sensible thing to do, even in good visibility, because apart from the man-overboard situation it brings familiarity with the compass and one never knows when visibility may deteriorate quickly.

If the compass course is known then the boat must be turned right round and steered on a reciprocal. This requires thought. If the boat was not actually being steered by compass, then the recent compass course should be deduced, which in many small craft may mean extracting the compass from its stowage below and shipping it in its mounting before making the turn. What I believe to be important in such a case is to maintain one's self-control and not to make the turn until one has some sure guidance about the correct reciprocal course. Success is going to depend on going back as near exactly as possible over the boat's track. To turn on to a guessed reciprocal, which may be 15 degrees off to one side or the other (and you don't know which) is obviously going to get you into a position where you just don't know where to turn next.

To keep a very sharp look-out, and to keep one's ears open must be obvious, but it is also pertinent to note the time at which the turn about is made, because logic demands that one sails back to the point corresponding to the last time the missing person was seen on board.

In a sailing boat it may be difficult to sail a reciprocal course. If the boat had been running then one will have to tack, and the skipper may decide that he can make a better job of it under power. But if he does choose (or is obliged) to sail, then turning to windward will require careful navigation and accurate timing of each tack if he is to hold close to the desired track. It all sounds very difficult, and it is likely to be so, yet if heads are kept clear there is a good chance of success, as has been proved in practice more than once.

KEEP HIM AFLOAT – AND IN VIEW

Very different is the situation where a person is seen to go over. The first thing is to get a lifebelt or some other buoyancy aid into the water and as near to him as possible, not only to give him support but also to mark the spot. One difficulty that arises is that some lightweight lifebuoys can blow away downwind very quickly, and that is why I think that every lifebuoy should be fitted with a drogue to slow its progress through the water.

There is also an incontrovertible argument for attaching to every lifebuoy an automatic electric lamp, since the very difficult business of spotting a man in a moving sea is made many times worse in the dark. And since a lamp may not be of much use by day, a suitable marker-buoy, with a flagstaff several feet high of bamboo or aluminium tube, is also provided by safety-conscious skippers.

Already we are somewhat removed from the conventional but over-simplified advice to 'throw him a lifebuoy'. And I believe one may have to take a further step and think whether that is good advice in any case. To *throw* a lifebuoy implies first that you have to extract the thing from some stowage where it is normally kept (and let's hope that its not in that highly decorative position in the main shrouds, but somewhere right at the helmsman's hand) and then that you have to throw it clear of backstay, ensign staff, pushpit or other obstructions. If the boat is moving at 6 knots she will be covering 10 feet in each second. Now I doubt if one can throw a lifebuoy much more than 20 feet in such circumstances, and even then there is a strong possibility that it will sail off on the wind and be carried just where you don't want it to go.

Still assuming a speed of 6 knots (*because* it works out conveniently at 10 feet a second) one may suppose that a quick-release stowage that allows the helmsman to drop the lifebuoy over the stern may be better than any attempt to throw it. If the helmsman has been drilled in what he has to do there is a fair chance that he will release the buoy in a second or two. It would then be in the water at the stern of the boat at very nearly the same time as a man who had fallen over from a point on deck 10 or 20 feet forward. Even if the man should fall off the transom of the boat a buoy released from the same point in the first second will probably be as near to him as one which is thrown three or four later.

All this is very arguable, but it bears thinking about, especially because lifebuoys on yachts are rarely arranged for a quick *drop* into the water. (By contrast, this is a common arrangement on ships.) This lack of lifebuoy release on many

47

yachts is only one aspect of the mental limitations of many yacht designers who seem to think that it is no part of their business to design safety installations, or even a housing for the steering compass, because such items are listed as 'optional extras'. I doubt if the same attitude would be regarded as good practice in other branches of engineering design, and one can only hope that things will gradually change. Just as an architect designing a block of flats must think of a fire-escape and other safety provisions, so should the naval architect think how he can help a man who goes overboard to get back again. Good marine design does, of course take into account such safety matters as fuel or electrical installations, and the lifelines and rails that help to keep a man on board, but the convention is to stop at that.

So it is that each owner or skipper must make up his own mind on these matters, using his eyes to see what others have done. No general methods can be laid down, but the aim is always to have lifebuoys in a place easy of access and stowed in such a way that they can be released on the instant.

Although the lifebuoy is universally used, it is possible that better devices could be devised with a bit of thought. For example, a string of floats, bent to a line perhaps 50 feet long at intervals of 10 feet and with a lifebuoy at the end would prove more effective. In the first place it would give the victim a greater chance of catching the line somewhere, and then with temporary support from one or more of the floats he could work the lifebuoy towards him. And it would give the crew of the returning yacht a much better chance in their turn of hooking the line at some point, after which it would be just a matter of drawing the man in. With floats of 8 inches diameter (say 20 cm, to make the arithmetic easy) each would have a volume of something over 4,000 millilitres, giving a buoyancy of 4 kilograms, or rather more than $8\frac{1}{2}$ lb. Yet the string of floats could be housed in a plastic tube of little over 8 inches in diameter and less than 3 feet in length. The lifebuoy, with its drogue would go into the water first, and as the yacht sailed on the float-line would be drawn from the tube and deployed across the sea.

Such a device sounds cumbersome, and requires to be proved in practice, but experiments I have made indicate that it is perfectly feasible. The two obvious risks are of a snarl-up in the line (it must be properly packed) and of catching it in one's propeller on the pick-up run. Fortunately one can get line (polypropylene for example) which floats, and flotation is in any case required for this purpose so that it can easily be seen and retrieved.

Quite apart from any fanciful ideas of mine on the subject, there is a choice to be made between the ring and horseshoe type of lifebuoy. The horseshoe seems most popular nowadays, and for most people it is the easier to get into. Likewise it is easier to come out of again, especially if one is getting tired. Therefore it seems sensible to fit a short line with a springhook that can be clipped across to close the mouth of the U when the wearer is inside.

In fact the old ring lifebelt is not so hard to get into if it is done the right way, and if the ring is large enough. One has to bring the ring in front of the face, grasp the edge with two hands and then twist the thing up and over so that it falls back over the head like a quoit falling over a peg at a hoop-la stall. The arms are then brought up, through and over, more or less in continuation of the same movement. It is not too hard if you know how, *if* you have practised it on bathing days, if you are not wearing excessively bulky clothing, and if the ring is big enough. The full-sized ring is 30 inches in diameter (760 mm), but smaller ones of 24 inches and even less are sold for yachts and these could cause trouble. Either kind could be troublesome to the guest who has not been instructed how it should be done.

Buoyant cushions, with roped edges which provide a hand-hold are a perfectly sensible thing to have in the cockpit. They do not fulfil the role of a lifebelt, but anything that can give temporary support and confidence to a man in the water is worth having. Even if one does have two lifebuoys on board

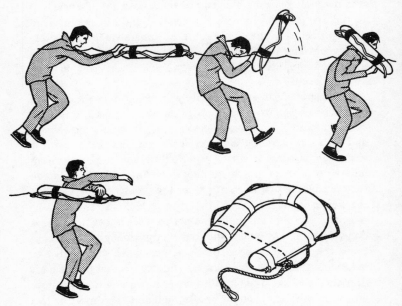

Getting into a circular lifebuoy requires a cool head – and practice. It is something that should be practised regularly on bathing days (when you also have the opportunity to find out whether your lifebuoy is big enough). The horseshoe pattern is easier to enter, and likewise easy to slip out of; so it is sensible to splice on a short length of line with a spring clip to close the mouth.

one would not want to throw them over simultaneously. One or two floating cushions give the man in the water an extra chance, and also help to mark the spot, which is extremely important.

There are also some useful proprietary gadgets. Dunlop make a pack containing a rubber quoit, which is easy to throw with some accuracy, attached to a length of light but strong line which is packed in such a way that it will run out easily. I feel that this gadget is best used from something stationary – a quayside, or a boat which is not making way. If thrown from a boat making 6 knots it would probably be jerked out of the hand of the poor chap, even if he did manage to grab it.

Then there is a cricket-ball sized pack, containing a self-inflating plastic bladder. Easy to throw and aim, but very likely to drift rapidly downwind when it inflates itself on the water. I shall have more to say about personal buoyancy gear in Chapter 12. In a sense there is no harm in having all the gear – if money is no object. But money usually is an object, so it becomes a matter of sorting out one's priorities. Moreover, the more gear one has the more important it will be to keep a cool head and to think which item is to be used for which situation. And that of course brings us to the nub of the matter, which is the need to keep a cool head in what is a very alarming and un-nerving situation. Haste in small boats very often leads to worse troubles, such as fouling one's own propeller with a line, or dismasting a sailing boat by a too-rapid gybe. That sort of thing is going to be no help at all in one's rescue plans.

One very good piece of rescue apparatus is the human swimmer. But that is something which implies a sizeable crew, which would make the whole process easier anyway. Never-theless, if a strong swimmer is available, who can put on a buoyancy waistcoat and a pair of frog-flippers and then enter the water deliberately, he should be able to make a personal delivery of a lifebuoy and line to the victim.

MANOEUVRING TO PICK HIM UP

A reader may observe that I am still perversely approaching the whole subject in reverse order, but now we come to the actual moment at which it all begins, when the cry of 'man over-board' is given by anyone (and everyone) who sees it happen and is repeated until all on board can have no doubt about it.

We assume that there is somebody at the helm, though the most dangerous times of all will be when the vessel is under the control of some kind of automatic steering device. (In this case there must very quickly be a living helmsman in charge.) The first consideration is to know the whereabouts of the man in the water, which means that somebody must keep him in sight. If the helmsman is the only chap left on board then he must somehow manage to do that as well as everything else. If there is a second person aboard he must watch the victim, but even so he is likely to have other duties as well. For example, in a sailing boat it will probably be necessary to gybe, but that involves attention to the main sheet, to the headsail sheets (and there may be more than one headsail), and possibly to runner backstays in some types of rig. And if the boat is carrying a spinnaker ... well in my view she has no right to be carrying such a sail unless she has an ample crew of able-bodied and competent people.

Incidentally, the problem of locating the victim is eased if visible floats, buoys and the like are known to be near him, or if he is known to be actually hanging on to something visible – it is the human head which disappears so easily if there is any sea running. But so long as the helmsman can see the victim, or can be directed towards him, his only remaining problem is to get the boat there in the shortest possible time. In a motor cruiser or a vessel under power with her sails set in light winds the problem is not too great. The turn may be made either way, though visibility from the helm may be a governing factor especially from a wheelhouse with an offset wheel. Otherwise it seems best to turn downwind because that will result in an upwind approach to the victim, which is likely to give better control.

Under power great care must be taken to avoid the possibility of causing injury with a propeller, and since it may be impracticable to stop the engine(s) precisely at the right moment it will be better to come up to leeward of the man. In that position the greater windage of the boat will tend to take her away from him, and although a parting is not what is really desired it will be better than having the boat blow down on top of him. Motor cruisers, with their generous top-hamper and rather parsimonious underwater areas, tend to make a rapid drift downwind.

In a sailing vessel the classical manoeuvre is also to turn downwind – to gybe in other words. 'Gybe immediately' is what many of us have engraved on our hearts, but a moment's reflection may well be repaid – especially if it is based on experience gained in practising. There are some courses on which a gybe must be the answer, but it is not the necessary manoeuvre for all courses as some books suggest. For example if the boat is running straight downwind she may turn either way for she must harden sheets and come close-hauled to sail back again. To gybe in such a case may be the wrong thing to do solely because it is a violent manoeuvre which may cause damage to gear or even people if the wind is strong.

It is because the object is to approach the man from a downwind position, that a gybe is normally the necessary action when the boat is sailing close-hauled. It is evident that to luff up and go on to the other tack effectively changes nothing – you are still beating away from the man, but on the other tack, and you are still left with the need to get downwind of him.

53

On a reach or a broad reach the usual answer will be to gybe, though other solutions are possible, depending on the agility of the boat herself and the exact point of sailing. In a boat which has a very small turning circle it may be possible to luff up and tack without changing the headsail sheet. Thus, the headsail will be aback and the boat will be hove-to. From this position it may be possible, with adjustment of the main sheet, to bring her back to the required position at a well controlled speed.

The beauty of this method, where it works, is that it can actually be quicker than gybing, that it is easier for the single-hander because no attention is required to the headsail sheets, and that the boat is moving slowly and under good control as she approaches the man. Now I expect that experienced skippers will want to protest, and I can say that I too protested when I was first introduced to it by Mr. Dove-Dixon while on a trial sail in a *Westerly Pageant*. But I at once put it to the test, using a fender-overboard rather than either of we too middle-aged gents (in any case, it was December, and snowing at the time), and after several timed tests I was convinced. In that particular boat, with her very short turning radius, luffing to back the headsail was a quicker way of getting back to the drifting fender than gybing. I have since tried the same procedure on other boats and can confirm that the *Pageant* is not unique. But as you might expect I can also say that more ponderous craft are not suited to this technique. Once again it comes down to the fact that experiment and practice are necessary so that each skipper can find out the best drill for his own boat.

Now it is very nice if you can arrive at your man with the boat virtually hove-to. But if you are beating back under sail then there will come a point when the sheets must be let fly so that the boat can carry her way until she comes to a stop at

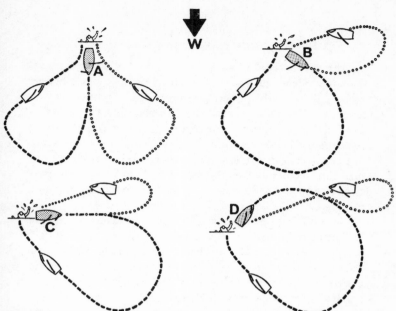

'Man overboard!' And though most text-books say that a gybe is the invariable manoeuvre to get back to him, that may not always be so. At **A**, the incident occurs while the boat is running with mainsail boomed out to port and there are two possible routes back, of which only one involves a gybe. It may be safer not to gybe in heavy weather, but putting the helm down and hardening in the main also involves more work with the headsail sheet . . . it's worth thinking about it.

At **B**, on a broad reach, a gybe is a sure way of getting back in the right on-the-wind attitude. But a very handy boat may be luffed through the wind without shifting the headsail sheet, so as to be hove-to. It is then possible to fore-reach slowly towards the victim. For a single-hander this is a more controlled manoeuvre than a gybe.

Similar considerations apply at **C**, when the sequence starts from a reach. But when close-hauled, as at **D**, the luff-up and heave-to technique is not likely to be practicable, unless you bear away first. *The only way to find the right method for a particular boat is to try them all.* It is worth timing both routes back if there are alternatives.

55

just the right place. In theory that requires nothing more than the same judgement that is required for picking up a mooring under sail, but with any sort of sea running judgement may be overtaxed. Then one may fall short, so that the boat falls off to leeward, leaving no choice but to gybe around and start all over again. A preferable error, in my view, would be to arrive too fast and overshoot. At least that gives control, and though you may carry your way past the man you should be able to pass close to him and to stream a long line over the stern which he can grab.

Since beating up requires judgement and takes time it may well be better to start the engine and do it under power. In light weather the sails may then be left to fend for themselves, though if hands are available to keep them quiet it will avoid the risk of further accidents due to flogging canvas and sheets, and help to promote an atmosphere of calm and order on board. Obviously that is only second priority to the main work of the crew, which is to prepare boathook and heaving line to bridge any gap that may remain between boat and man when the helmsman has done his best.

It is a situation full of ifs and buts, and I do not offer any simple clear-cut solution which is as easy to remember as the long-publicised rule 'always gybe at once'. I don't believe that to be right. The only sound advice is to think about it, then practise, think some more, and then practise again.

If, at the end of all this the day should come when one fishes a chap out of the water, one cannot necessarily be sure that that will be the end of the trouble. Much depends on the water temperature and the length of time the man has been in it, for although drowning may have been averted death can still follow after rescue. That can happen as a result of heat loss which cools the body to a dangerously low temperature. If the victim comes back on board in an obviously fit condition after a short immersion then there's no need to worry; but if he is shivery, seems unable to see, hear or speak normally, has cramp, or seems in any way other than his normal self, then very great care must be taken in his treatment. And this is a subject which will conveniently make another chapter.

4. Artificial Respiration and Aftercare

The modern method of artificial respiration is to use your own lungs to pump air into those of the victim. It is simple to do and easy to understand – far more so than any of the older methods. The drill is as follows:

Lay the man on his back.

Clear his mouth of anything that may be obstructing, and remove false teeth.

Tilt the head back by pressing the forehead with one hand while the other provides support under the nape of the neck.

Now use one hand to hold the forehead back while its fingers pinch his nostrils to close his nose, and with the other hand control his jaw so that the mouth is sufficiently opened to mate with your own. Make sure his tongue has not dropped back to block the throat.

Take a deep breath, open your mouth wide and seal your lips around his.

Exhale into his lungs until they are filled.

Remove your mouth and watch his chest fall. Then repeat.

In principle the system is very simple, but like everything

else it is better to practise. Some additional comments must be made. In the first place speed is important, and if it seems necessary the treatment can be begun in the water. Likewise, if it is not possible to lay him out flat in the small cockpit of a boat just adopt the best possible position that will allow the lungs to expand.

If for any reason his mouth cannot be used (if it were injured, say) the air can be delivered through his nose.

It is important to remember that his lungs may not be so big as yours, so don't overdo it – and take special care with infants and children – it is easy to do serious harm to their lungs by over-inflation.

With babies and infants it may be more practical to engulf both nose and mouth with your own. And though smaller 'doses' will be required they will be needed more frequently – at about 3-second intervals, whereas the period for an adult would be 5 or 6 seconds.

After inflating the lungs five or six times the patient should begin to look better, if his heart is working, for oxygen supplied to his lungs will now be circulating in his blood to give him a better colour. But if you think he still looks grey it will be necessary to try and stimulate the heart. If you are alone it will mean that you must temporarily abandon the insufflation, but if two people are available both activities can continue in parallel.

HEART MASSAGE

Raise the legs above the level of the chest to help blood to run towards the heart.

Thump his breastbone hard with your fist.

Start pressing the breastbone rhythmically at a rate of about once a second. If single-handed, do that about fifteen times before going back to forced respiration. Then after five lung inflations go back to heart massage and continue alternating like this until you either achieve success or until *rigor mortis* is evident – i.e. until his muscles stiffen.

Some comments. The thump on the breastbone sounds a bit crude – in fact it is crude, rather like shaking a watch to set it going, but it can be an effective method for the human ticker too. The rhythmical compression of the breastbone is not such a simple matter as it sounds for it requires quite a high pressure to bend the bone inward by the inch (or perhaps a little more) that is required. Yet one must not go so far as to fracture a rib. It is the breastbone on which you must press, though, and not the ribs.

EFFECTS OF COLD

One danger that is not widely understood is that of hypothermia – a lowering of the body temperature due to immersion in cold water. As I said in the preceding chapter, if the rescued person needs no artificial respiration or heart massage, but seems shivery, unable to see, hear or speak properly, or not in normal control of himself, then hypothermia must be considered likely.

One must not make the mistake of trying to warm him up rapidly, but at the same time any further loss of heat must be prevented. Time is not wasted in removing or changing the victim's wet clothing, but he must be wrapped up and protected from the wind. This does not mean merely putting a blanket over him as he lies on a berth – it means cocooning so that all possible routes for heat loss are sealed off.

Sugar, golden syrup, sweetened condensed milk and other easily-taken forms of sugar can be given, but do not give hot drinks at this stage, nor a hot-water bottle. Sudden heating may prove fatal. Likewise this is not the time for a cheering tot of grog – not for the patient at any rate. It is a matter of 'cocoon and wait' – unless artificial respiration or heart massage becomes necessary, of course.

I will leave it at that, since I have no intention of turning this into a treatise on first aid, nor the qualifications to do it. Good books are available in plenty. But it may be as well to point out that drowning, which follows the entry of water into the lungs, is a process that happens very rapidly. Death follows not from the lack of air and oxygen, but from an imbalance in the body's fluids. By the process of osmosis water is transferred through the lung walls, to or from the remainder of the body. If salt water enters the lungs the body loses water and its fluid becomes too saline. On the other hand, if fresh water gets into the lungs it diffuses through into the blood stream and dilutes it, so lowering the body's salinity. Either process is fatal, and in practice irreversible. The point seems worth making because I have come across otherwise well-informed people who suppose that one of the objects of artificial respiration and external cardiac massage was to 'get the water out of the lungs'.

It is sensible to have 'potted' instructions on a card where it can be quickly found. Such sheets are obtainable from the Royal Life Saving Society, 14 Devonshire Street, Portland Place, London W.1., the Royal Society for the Prevention of Accidents, 1 Grosvenor Crescent, London S.W.1, and the St John Ambulance Society and the British Red Cross, among others.

IN REAL LIFE

I suspect that to many people there is an air of unreality about these life-saving drills, as if they were just a way of keeping

Boy Scouts occupied on a wet afternoon. But just to show what they can mean in real life, here is just one paragraph extracted from the annual report (1970) of the Chief Inspector of H.M. Coastguard. Mr Ronan, an Auxiliary Coastguard had asked for help from Station Officer Timothy in retrieving a 'body' from the sea . . .

By this time Mr Ronan had hauled the body of an elderly man on board his speedboat and Mr Timothy, on arrival of the boat alongside the slipway boarded her and immediately commenced Mouth to Mouth resuscitation, and *after five minutes had elapsed* (my italics – D.D.) the man commenced to gurgle and vomited. A helper who had arrived on the scene informed Mr Timothy that there was no heart beat and he was given cardiac resuscitation which proved successful. Ambulance men then arrived and took over.

5. Fire and Explosion

Newspaper reports alone must be enough to make anyone aware that fire and explosion take their toll of boats each year, and although I have no national statistics it would seem that when one goes boating one has at least as much chance of being blown up as of being drowned.

Serious fires on boats are often preceded by an explosion, but in either case it will usually be found that either petrol or bottled gas is involved. Minor fires may come from a variety of causes – from careless handling of cigarettes to dropping paraffin lamps or overheated frying fat. But in the serious ones, and for explosions in particular, petrol or bottled gas are likely to be essential components.

That is because these are the only two things customarily carried on board a boat which are likely to go up *'whoosh'*. Paraffin burns, and so does diesel oil, but neither burns explosively unless it is first heated well above ordinary atmospheric temperatures. Methylated spirit (also known as industrial alcohol) is often carried, either for starting paraffin cookers and lamps, or as a principal cooking fuel. And meths, which vaporises easily, will explode, but it is such a feeble little *plop* that nothing much is to be feared from it.

One other explosive vapour may regularly be present, and that is the hydrogen gas given off by a lead-acid battery while it is being charged. But although precautions must be taken, that gas is not a primary risk because hydrogen is so much lighter than air. Thus it floats rapidly upward, and if there is reasonable ventilation above the battery each molecule of hydrogen escapes up, up, and away as soon it slips out of the battery vent-hole.

BOTTLED-GAS INSTALLATION

But with bottled gas it is quite a different story. This gas, which is either butane or propane, or a mixture of the two, is much heavier than air. In consequence it runs down to the lowest level it can reach, just like water. *Just like water.* If one can get that picture of the invisible gas running down over a locker front and between cracks in floorboards just as if it were water one is already well fore-armed. It is difficult to accustom oneself to the thought of gas behaving in that way because we are mostly accustomed to kitchen gas which wafts away upward. But you can pour bottled gas from the bottle into a bucket until it fills over the brim and runs down on to the ground. And of course, if the ground is parched and cracked it will go on down, possibly to reappear some distance downhill.

Ordinary petrol fuel evaporates into a gas (or vapour) which is also heavier than air, and so runs downhill like liquid petrol. In passing it may be worth remarking that bottled gas is derived from petroleum and is therefore known in the trade as Liquefied Petroleum Gas, or LPG.

Either of these gases becomes dangerous in a boat because a boat is a watertight and gastight vessel. If you have a gas leak in a caravan, or a petrol leak in a car, then there is every chance that the vapour will escape downward and spread over the ground. In a boat that cannot happen, and if there is any leak in a gas system, or any spillage of petrol, one is very likely to have an accumulation of potentially explosive vapour in the bottom of the boat.

Whether these vapours will explode or simply burn when ignited depends on the proportion of gas to air, and that does not really concern us very much. What can be said is that most people's noses are able to detect the presence of LPG or petrol vapour at concentrations far too weak to cause an explosion. A smell is deliberately added to bottled gas for that purpose by the way, and a very useful protection it is too. But some people have a poor sense of smell, and there is in any case the chance that gas may leak down into the bilges without ever coming near your nose. Gas-detecting instruments are available to meet that case, at a price, though they are rarely found in cruising boats in the 'under-ten-ton' category.

But for most of us our defence will lie first in *care* – care about the standard and condition of our gas installation, and care in its use.

The first wise step with the installation is to keep it as simple as possible, and it is not a bad idea to limit it to cooking only. If that can be done, then you can get away with a single run of pipe from bottle to cooker, and there is obviously far less risk of a leak than there would be with an extensive circuit feeding water-heater, refrigerator, lights and some cabin heaters too. If such devices are desired, then they can be bought with thermocouple sensors fitted which will close the supply if the flame goes out. Even so, that still leaves the possibility of a leak somewhere along the supply line.

Without doubt the most popular installation is the simple, *bottle-line-cooker*. A good, but often impractical, place for the bottle is on deck, perhaps in a wooden casing with holes at the bottom so that any spilled gas can run out, across the deck and over the side. Many modern boats are built with a special gas-bottle locker above the waterline and with a drain-hole going out through the side of the boat. The locker must be gastight, but only up as far as the top of the bottle. There is no call for a gastight lid of course.

The line from the bottle should be of good quality annealed copper, or of neoprene rubber sold specifically for use with bottled gas and armoured with a woven wire sheath. Furthermore, one uses one's common sense to ensure that the pipe does not suffer any strain, or vibration or chafe which could harm it. Among other things that means having both the bottle and the cooker firmly restrained so that neither can move and so load the pipe.

Most people will carry a spare, full bottle of gas, and some like to keep both bottles connected to a T-junction pipe because the gas always runs out while you're cooking and it's so much easier to open one valve and close another than to change bottles. That's very nice, but it is important to have a non-return valve in each arm of the T, so that gas cannot escape when you do get around to replacing the empty bottle.

When replacing bottles always check for a leak by smearing soap and water (or detergent and water) over the joint while the gas-bottle valve is open, but keeping the cooker shut off. Many bottles do not need washers in their assembly, but make a metal-to-metal seal. If your particular make does require a washer it is worth finding out precisely what type of washer is correct and then laying in a supply. There was a time when I shared with many others, including some retail suppliers of gas bottles, the misapprehension that the washer which arrived with the bottle, sealed under the protective plastic cap, was the correct one to use for a connection. It was not. I consider myself lucky to have survived so well for so long before finding out what nobody in the trade had tried to tell me.

As it happens that type of bottle and assembly is not so widely used nowadays, but the principle remains the same:

unless one is quite sure, it is worth making a positive effort to find out.

A leak can also occur at the cooker tap. There is sometimes a gland through which the control rod from the visible knob reaches the valve. This can be tightened, like the gland in a stern tube, with the nut which is usually behind the faceplate.

CARE IN THE USE OF GAS – LADIES PLEASE NOTE

I say 'ladies please note', but I think that in practice most women are even more thoughtful about the danger of bottled gas than the men. So let us all note well, and so save ourselves from a nasty experience.

The main valve which is built in to the top of each gas bottle is about as reliable as any piece of mechanical equipment can be, so one sure way of avoiding a leak is to turn the gas off at the bottle whenever it is not in use. That is a fairly simple procedure on a boat which has a simple installation – just a bottle and a cooker. If all the members of the family are taught to be gas-conscious there will be some little voice piping up to remind you if you forget, and although it can be irritating at the time it is something of a satisfaction later on.

The second point on which to take care is to be sure that the flame does not go out. On many small craft the galley is near the main hatch, where there are plenty of draughts, and bottled gas does have rather a soft flame. Many gas cookers intended for boats and caravans have a two-position tap that clicks either to *full on*, or to *simmer*. The underlying idea is to discourage people from turning the flame right down to the lowest possible level, where it might too easily go out.

With the same object in view it is worth watching for any pan that might boil over and put the flame out. An event which would be a minor irritation with a gas cooker at home can be positively dangerous when you are using a gas which is heavier than air.

Given that the boat is being used regularly by the same family and that everybody understands what should be done, and why it should be done, then I don't think that there is very much to fear from the simplest gas installation on a small boat. A great many of the disasters which are reported in the daily press concern hire boats, where the situation is very different. Without doubt the hire company explains to each party just what they should do, and without doubt most people are sensible. But where hundreds of boats are involved, and each one has a different crew each week, one would expect that sooner or later some clot will come along . . .

With a more complex gas installation the situation is not so easy to manage. If there is a network of pipes running through the boat to supply refrigerator, water-heater, cabin-heaters and lamps, then there is no possibility of 'turning off at the bottle after every use'. My own choice would be to use electricity for all services other than cooking, but if for some reason gas is being used then I believe that it becomes essential to install a gas-detecting instrument.

VENTILATION

Unlike the old-fashioned town-gas, bottled gas is not in itself poisonous. Nevertheless it has a great appetite for oxygen and if it has to share the same supply as the human occupants of a cabin it is likely to 'win'. One might expect that if the cabin were sealed up the flame would go out when the oxygen became short, but unfortunately it is we who are likely to go out first. And as we lose consciousness the gas burner, starved of air, will begin to form poisonous carbon monoxide which might finish the job off . . .

The same consideration can apply with Tilley lamps, solid-fuel stoves and other devices that require air to burn. Fortunately most boats have sufficient natural (though often unintentional) ventilation to cope with this situation. Doors and hatches usually do not fit so well as those ashore, and there are ways for air to enter the cabin via the bilges and the cabin sole, or perhaps through lockers which have sensibly been provided with ventilation holes.

But it is a point to be watched, especially when one turns in for the night. That is a time when it is best to extinguish any devices which may compete with you and your family for the available oxygen.

PETROL-FUEL INSTALLATION

With petrol the objective is the same as it is with bottled gas – to prevent the accumulation of vapour in the bilges. That also embraces the need to avoid spills or leakages of liquid petrol which will quite quickly turn into a vapour which can explode if mixed with the right proportion of air. Obviously it is also important to avoid igniting liquid petrol!

This is not a book for yacht designers who must be presumed to know what precautions should be taken with petrol and gas installations. But neither designers nor builders are always infallible in practice, so it is up to each owner to check the installation on his own boat in the interests of his own safety.

Quite apart from the fact that there may have been a fault when the boat was delivered from the yard (I recall the case of a fuel pipe which ran above a red-hot exhaust pipe on to which it dripped petrol with most serious consequences for the owner and his wife) there is also the possibility that some subsequent alteration or addition may have been made without proper thought. Some piece of electrical equipment may perhaps have been installed in a position where it could receive petrol from a flooding carburettor.

The things to check begin with the fuel tank and its filler. The filler point should be in a position where an overflow will run over the ship's side into the water. That usually means that the filler must be outside the cockpit on a sidedeck.

A risk that is sometimes forgotten is that of the static spark which can jump between ship and filler hose when the two are at a different electrical potential. I will not attempt a description of how it happens that these separate electrical charges can occur, but there is no doubt that they do. Thus it is wise, before running the fuel, to bring the nozzle of the filler hose into contact with the flange of the fuel inlet on deck. If this fitting is not naturally in electrical circuit with the fuel tank itself, as may be the case where a length of rubber hose forms the connection, then a copper wire should be permanently fitted between the two. Thus, hose nozzle, filler, inlet and tank can be got to the same potential before fuel begins to flow.

The best installations have a filler pipe that runs to a point just above the bottom of the tank. This minimises stirring and splashing as the fuel goes in, and thus reduces vapour formation. It also reduces the (in any case slight) chance that static electrical charges may be formed inside the tank as a result of the agitation of the fuel. This ideal arrangement is rather rare, and in the small-volume tanks and the low-flow rates that are found with yachts the risk must be deemed to be negligible.

Gravity feed is best avoided where possible because of the evident risk that a ruptured fuel pipe will allow all the fuel to run away into the boat. A tank placed low in the boat, with pump feed to the engine is preferred by the best authorities. The fuel line to the engine will normally be of annealed copper

– that's to say relatively soft copper. With the passage of time and especially if under the influence of vibration, the copper will harden and become more likely to crack. There are two defences. The first, a counsel of perfection, is to remove the pipe and have it annealed. That excellent plan is seldom followed, I regret to say. The other defence is to sheath the pipe from one end to the other in plastic tubing, which must be gripped to the copper with stainless steel pipe clips at each end. The plastic tube (PVC) will protect the copper against chafe, and against the risk of somebody dumping a sharp object on it, and will also provide a line of defence against a leak. Nevertheless it will still be necessary to inspect it from time to time; if petrol is visible inside the plastic then you know what has happened.

Joints in the fuel pipe should be kept to the minimum and ordinary solder must not be used. They may be brazed, or they may be mechanical couplings of the screwed or compression type.

Visual inspection, plus the use of a modest amount of imagination, should reveal danger points. There was the case of a boat which was completely destroyed because an electric relay was fitted to a bulkhead immediately below a fuel filter. The man who fitted it there obviously lacked the perspicacity to see that if ever the fuel filter assembly should leak, petrol would drip on the relay. In fact that did ultimately happen, and the boat was burned out down to the waterline.

Following the fuel line along its course from tank to engine, one looks to be sure that it cannot be damaged by any foreseeable event, neither by the shifting of ballast, nor by the stowing of an anchor, nor by chafe where it passes through a bulkhead. (A protective outer sleeve of PVC will help there, of course.) Vibration at the engine end may cause unions to loosen, or may crack the pipe. Hence it is customary to put a couple of full loops or turns in the pipe, in the manner of a coilspring, to absorb such movement.

An obvious trap to be avoided is to have any sort of outlet tap or drain cock in the fuel line *en route* to the engine. Apart from the fact that the additional joints provide additional chances for leaks, there is the risk that the tap may be accidentally knocked open. Beware, too, of the spark-plug leads of the engine itself. As it becomes older the insulation on these leads grows less effective, and the high voltage will send sparks across to nearby parts of the engine. One night many years ago I took the hatch cover off my engine as we were motoring out of the harbour and was shocked to see bright little sparks jumping from the high-tension lead to the brass body of the carburettor float-chamber! That shows the value of a night inspection, and emphasises the need to route H.T. leads well clear of metal work.

The carburettor itself should have a protective gauze, or flame arrester, fitted over the air intake against the risk of spitting back, and below it there should be a small trough or bowl to collect any spilled petrol. The petrol may come from flooding while starting or from a sticking float-chamber needle. The collecting trough must be covered with wire gauze, to act in the manner of the miner's safety lamp mesh which we remember from our schooldays.

It is necessary to draw my line somewhere. Perhaps one can simply urge owners to look at their petrol system with the same suspicion that they would give a ticking bomb. Try to picture what could possibly happen, knowing that if it *can*, it *will*.

CARE IN FUELLING WITH PETROL:
ALL TO NOTE PLEASE

Yes, the ladies too, for when petrol is being taken on board all naked lights must be extinguished. So out goes the cooker, plus any paraffin lamp or cigarette that may be burning. Furthermore, during the fuelling process, and for five minutes or so after it is finished, no switch should be actuated for fear that it will cause a spark. Switches do create sparks, even though one does not normally see them. The one exception to this rule about switches concerns those which are known to be in flame-proof boxes, designed to be safe. Such a switch would be associated with an engine compartment ventilating fan, which is evidently a proper thing to be used while fuelling.

A good rule with both petrol and gas is to be very suspicious. If the engine will not start, don't go on pressing the starter switch – perhaps a fuel connection has come loose so that the petrol is running into the bilge instead of into the carburettor. If that should be the case then it will explain the engine's failure to start. But it also means that a potentially explosive mixture is building up below your feet, and the next time you try to work the starter a spark from the motor may initiate the big bang.

It is regrettable that any honest discussion about risks such as these must make mention of some rather gruesome facts, but it is important to emphasise how powerful a petrol-vapour explosion can be. It usually blows the decks off, and the people on board over the side and into the water. It has also been known to blow the transom off the stern of the boat and the planks out of the bow. It is just like an explosion of dynamite, gelignite or the like (at least if there is any subtle difference I don't think it is of a kind likely to worry the victim!)

Other fire risks associated with the engine can be minimised by fairly simple checks. The exhaust pipe for example; often it is water-jacketed or cooled by water mixed with the exhaust

73

gases, but in some boats it can become very hot. So one looks to see that it does not pass too close to any woodwork, especially painted woodwork. Nor must there be any chance that fuels, white spirit or paint or even lubricating oil can spill on to it when the boat pitches and rolls at sea. Sails and oilskins must be kept clear – in fact one uses a bit of common sense.

ELECTRICS

Then the battery. I have already mentioned the chance of igniting hydrogen gas if the battery is not adequately ventilated. Probably a more serious risk is that of some metal object falling across the terminals of the battery and causing a direct short-circuit. I recall seeing one boat in which a spare can of petrol was precariously propped in a position where it could easily have fallen across the terminals of a battery below. That was a perfect recipe for disaster. Then again, there is always the person who has a berth alongside in a marina, with a supply of mains electricity. That provides him with the means to use a trickle charger, which is very convenient – until he goes away for a few days and forgets to disconnect. After the battery is fully charged it boils dry, then overheats and bursts into flames, with the probable loss of a boat. Forethought is the need.

The internal electrical system of a boat, even though it may be only at 12 volts, is a potential source of fire. A short circuit or a wire too small for the current it is being asked to carry, may quickly set fire to woodwork or furnishings. One must therefore look out for signs of chafe in wires, or for the odd screw that may have pierced the insulation. It's easily done – perhaps in fitting up a mirror or the like, one can drive a screw through a bulkhead or a shelf and into an electric lead without knowing it. Equally, wiring which was of adequate size for the job it was expected to do when the boat was built, may become overloaded because successive owners have added extra appliances to the outlet end without giving thought to the relation between the size of wire and the total current it may have to carry.

Apart from these rather recondite sources of fire there are all the usual 'domestic' things, such as carelessly dropped matches, smoking in bed, a tea towel too near the stove and so forth. On a boat they are more serious than at home because you are in a confined space and may not be able to run away, nor is it likely that you will be able to call the fire brigade to your help. Furthermore boats are most commonly built of inflammable material.

One need not stress that wood burns, but it is worth saying a word or two about 'fibreglass', because people know that glass does not burn. But the boats which are commonly called 'fibreglass' are in fact made of polyester resin, and the glass fibre is simply a reinforcement for the plastic. The resin in fact burns *very* well, and usually even more of a fibreglass boat is destroyed in a fire than of a wooden boat. Not that it makes much difference because either kind is very likely to be burned beyond salving.

But if a fire should start we must be prepared to put it out; and that is a subject which needs a chapter to itself.

6. When You Must Be
Your Own Fireman

Fire-fighting is a specialised business, requiring special knowledge and thorough training. The same may be said of navigation, and the other activities that we amateur boating enthusiasts must dabble in. We have to do the best we can as painters, riggers and shipwrights – and we have to cook, look after the children and tend the engine when it goes wrong.

Obviously we cannot tackle all these jobs in precisely the same way that the professionals would do it. We have to find our own methods, and very often the professionals, I believe, would do it our way if they found themselves in our shoes.

The greatest weakness of the amateur fire-fighter is that he is not likely to have had any practice. Even if he *has* had a go with a fire extinguisher on something easy – his bonfire, or a tray of burning petrol, he is hardly likely to have set fire to his boat just to see what happens ... And a boat fire can be a particularly awkward one to deal with. We have large quantities of inflammable material packed closely into a small space, and to make it worse there is a volume under the cockpit and cabin floors (the 'soles' in nautical language) which is likely to contain oil and fuel floating on water. Down there the timber may be steeped in oil that has been spilled over the years, and at the worst there may be an accumulation of spilled petrol or petrol vapour, or bottled cooking gas.

There are also the fires of electric origin. But a family boat usually has a low voltage supply (6, 12 or 24 volt) so that we don't have any fear of electrocution. Thus a fire of electrical origin does not require special treatment, which is a simplification.

NON-FUEL FIRES

So what we have in practice is two kinds of fire, needing two kinds of extinguishant. The first kind is relatively simple because it involves ordinary materials – wood, wool, newspapers, cooking fat and the like. This kind of fire can be dealt with in two main ways, either by dousing with water, or by stifling under a blanket. *Water* is by far the best fire extinguishant for fires other than those involving engine fuels or cooking fat. If, for example, someone should drop a cigarette into a locker full of cotton sails, then water will be a far better extinguishant than the best chemical device you can buy. Its merit lies in the fact that it can soak the burning mass right through, and cool it down. And usually there is plenty of water near a boat.

The same would apply to something like a burning sleeping bag. Like as not the fire has started somewhere within, and there has been a long period of smouldering with a steady increase of internal heat before flames suddenly burst out. In such a case it is not enough to extinguish the flames on the surface – somehow the whole mass of the material must be cooled, and any smouldering in the inner core must be stopped, or else it will burst into flames once again. Water is the perfect answer; except that you finish up with a wet berth.

A layer of burning fat in a frying pan is a different matter. Smother it with a cloth – a damp tea-towel, your oilskin jacket or anything else that comes to hand – and you will stop the fire by depriving it of oxygen. Unless you are foolish enough to leave the gas-ring alight beneath it, all that is then necessary is

77

to leave it smothered for a few moments to cool down, and there is no reason to fear re-ignition. A fine technical sounding term, 're-ignition', but one worth remembering because if ever you extinguish a fire it is necessary to be on guard against the chance that it will start up again. One must make quite sure that the materials involved have cooled right down before one can relax.

Some yacht chandlers sell asbestos fire blankets, complete with container, and this is a worthwhile piece of equipment to have in any boat which is big enough to stow it. The blanket is kept rolled up in its container – an open-ended tube – from which you can pull it instantly.

TACKLING A FUEL FIRE IN THE BILGE: WHAT KIND OF EXTINGUISHER?

We now come to the point where I must ask the reader to be good enough to bear with me while I parade various propositions and arguments concerning the way in which one should tackle what we may conveniently call 'bilge fires'. I have read many articles, and some books, and have sat through lectures, in which simple categorical statements about fire-fighting on yachts were made. But, and it is a 'but' which must be important to us all, I have not been convinced by what is generally said. It is not in fact a simple problem that we face.

At this point I must confess that I have never had to face a fire on my own boat. On the other hand, I have collected information from those who have, and their experiences broadly confirm what I believe to be the common fallacy about fire-fighting on small boats. So I shall put forward what may be called the conventional ideas as well as my own, and leave each to decide what is best for his particular boat.

The type of boat, her engine installation and other factors

relevant to each case are very important, and what suits one case may not suit another. That we shall see as we proceed.

Right, then, let's get on with it.

As most people will know, one cannot fight petrol, diesel or lubricating oil fires with water. The burning fuel floats on top of the water, and tends to be spread around by the splashing of the water as it arrives. So the simple methods that are used for wood and cloth fires must give way to special equipment – in other words some kind of proprietary fire extinguisher. We can immediately eliminate the CTC extinguisher for a start. The brass-bodied, plunger-pump type of extinguisher, containing carbon tetrachloride, was at one time quite widely supplied for use in boats, and these lethal little gadgets must still be hanging on many a bulkhead. But this compound is very toxic, and not a very good extinguishant. It is true that CTC can be used to clean clothing, but most people who have knowledge would advise that, because of its toxicity, it should be dumped where it can do no harm to human or animal life. In short, do not allow any CTC on board, and if you do have one of those brass-pump devices, empty the CTC and refill with water. (This, by the way, is not just a bee in my personal bonnet. It is a view on which I don't think there is any division of opinion.)

With CTC out of the way we can turn to the possible types of fire-extinguishant that can be used aboard a boat. They are:

Dry powder

Foam

Carbon dioxide

BCF liquid/vapour

Any of these will extinguish a fire very effectively *if it can reach the burning surface*. If one has petrol or fuel oil burning in the bilges of the boat it may or may not be floating on water, but in either case the fire will be on the surface of the fuel. So this is a different situation from the deep-seated fire in a bundle of sails. Furthermore, if this fuel fire gets a few minutes to its own devices it will begin to set light to timber or resin which is nearby. These will also burn on the surface.

There we have the picture of the fire we are trying to tackle – it is beneath the engine; under the cabin seating, below the galley cooker; around the corner behind the oilskin locker; and in any case beneath the cabin or cockpit soles – or beneath both. So it has always seemed to me that the *principle problem we face is to get the extinguishant to the fire.*

As far as I am concerned that rules out **dry powder**, which is the choice of the Home Office Committee which wrote a report on this subject some years ago (*Fire Precautions in Pleasure Craft*, HMSO). And that's a pity, because the virtues of dry powder (mainly bicarbonate of soda) which attracted the officials cannot be denied. It is harmless to people and is a good extinguishant. But if you cannot project it round those corners to reach the fire then I think that that is the end of the matter. Experiments I made some years ago with small fires in baffled compartments to simulate the maze of structure in a boat convinced me that dry powder projected from an extinguisher will *not* flow round corners. Since then I have had confirmation from one boat owner who had to try it for real. There is one other possible drawback to dry powder, though it is overcome in the better quality extinguishers, and that is that the grains may compact into a more or less solid mass over a period of time, helped by the settling effect of prolonged exposure to engine vibrations. Thus there is a *chance* that an extinguisher, though still full, may not work when you want it.

Foam, given time, would fill an under-floor space. You could poke the nozzle down through a small hole in the cockpit sole, and gradually all the empty spaces below would fill up. But the problem with foam-making apparatus is its bulk, and I don't think many people with boats even of 10 tons could find space for it. Furthermore, it is heavy, and that is a very pertinent point when it comes, as it may, to manoeuvring the apparatus while the boat is rolling and you are trying to work fast.

Both **carbon dioxide** and **BCF** are gases, and they are a better bet because they will migrate through the spaces that we are concerned with. Because they are gases there is also a chance that they may be drawn along towards the flames by the natural draught that any fire creates to feed itself. Well, just a *chance*.

Of the two, BCF is the better extinguishant, so you need less of it to do a given job. BCF offers a further space and weight advantage because carbon dioxide has to be stored at a much higher pressure. It is one of BCF's valuable qualities that it can be liquefied at ordinary temperatures by a pressure of about 20 lb to the square inch. When you press the button to open the valve it changes to gas (i.e. 'vapour') as it leaves the nozzle. Very convenient. Carbon dioxide behaves in the same way, but it has to be stored at a pressure of 600 lb to the square inch, which is not convenient because it requires stouter, heavier bottles.

Putting these facts into the context of the stowage space available in a small boat, there is no doubt that as far as the extinguishing of a fire is concerned, BCF is the better stuff to choose. But now we come to the area where my own practice departs from the Home Office advice, because the official pamphlet simply says that 'vaporising liquids are not recommended for use in private pleasure craft'. That blanket veto also rules out a number of other compounds along with BCF – compounds such as methyl bromide, chlorobromethane, and others which we can all agree should definitely not be used on boats because they are harmful to both the materials of which the boat is built and to the people on board. So they can be forgotten, for among the vaporising liquids it is BCF (bromochlorodifluoromethane) or nothing.

Now although BCF in sufficient concentration is harmful to human beings I don't think that we need fear it in ordinary circumstances. Even a sudden and total leak of your extinguisher into your cabin could not achieve a concentration of the gas sufficient to poison you – in the usual sense of the word. From calculations I have made I do not think it could even reach the level where you would begin to feel 'wuzzy', and so fail to get up and go into the fresh air. That is an important consideration, of course, because although one would normally realise that something had happened and make for fresh air, there is the chance of a leak while you are asleep. As I keep a small BCF extinguisher near my berth, against the chance of a night fire, I was very conscious of that danger. That is why I sought out the best figures that I could get from ICI's medical researchers and the Fire Research Station as a basis for a bit of simple arithmetic. To cut the matter short, I am now confident that there is no need for any alarm on that point.

There are risks in everything. Even carbon dioxide can be dangerous in a sufficient concentration. So for that matter can the water vapour that may saturate the air if enough water is poured on a hot enough fire. It is a matter of reasonably likely situations.

When it comes to the deliberate discharge of a BCF extinguisher then I think that the risk is even less. One is then aware of what one is doing, and unless somebody is going to shut himself up in the loo and let off the whole barrel-full in there, we shall have nothing to worry about. EXCEPT that when BCF comes into contact with a hot fire other and much more unpleasant compounds are formed. These are acid gases which are both toxic and irritating, and I believe that they must have been the main worry to the Home Office committee. But they must have had in mind the needs of boats much bigger than I suppose readers of this book to own. They would have to consider craft with several cabins, possibly even several decks, and corridors and suchlike. In that sort of boat you could very well have a situation where people were sleeping in some cabins while extinguishers were going off (perhaps automatically) in an engine room somewhere below. There would be the likelihood that some of these nasty acid gases would find their way into the cabins where people were sleeping. A serious point.

But in my boat the situation is very different. She is quite small, the hatches are large in relation to the internal volume, and there is no possibility of anybody being more than twenty feet away from anybody else. If we had a fire anywhere on board we should all know about it virtually at the same moment, and we should all get out on deck or into the cockpit. Indeed the only thing that might stop us would be that the fire itself was in the way. In that case, as in all others, the main aim would be to get the fire out as quickly as possible, and the sooner it is out the sooner the gas fumes will come to an end. I believe that many small craft and their crews must be very much the same.

Others may take a different view. They may be willing to face the bulk of the heavier carbon dioxide equipment. They may have boats whose arrangement makes it feasible to bring dry powder to the seat of any likely fire. It is an important matter on which we must all make up our own minds, and unfortunately there is no gaseous extinguishant available which is completely free of undesirable side-effects – if there were there would be no problem. As it is I find myself forced to the conclusion that I must use BCF for inaccessible fires, though I also carry a powder extinguisher which I would use when possible.

One point in BCF's favour is that it evaporates quickly. For that reason it does not stay around long enough to harm the polyester resin of a 'fibreglass' boat.

HOW MANY EXTINGUISHERS MUST ONE HAVE?

Having dealt at some length with the type of extinguishant, I must now deploy some points of view on the number and type of 'appliances' one should carry on board. Here again, I believe that you must take full account of the particular boat you have in view, and of the conditions aboard that particular boat. It is wise to assume that a fire may start at any point in the boat, and that you may be at any point when that happens. You could be in the cabin, and the fire could bar your way aft to the cockpit – or *vice versa*. One can think out permutations that correspond to the topography of one's own boat, always remembering the law propounded by the famed Professor Sodde who stated that things tend to happen in the most awkward and inconvenient manner!

Evidently you don't want to find yourself in a situation where the fire is between you and the extinguisher. And the logical conclusion is to opt for a large number of small and cheap devices scattered through the boat, so that there is always one within arm's reach. Or in another boat it might be possible to find a practical solution with just a couple of 3 lb or 5 lb bottles strategically placed.

A difficulty with the 'many and small' philosophy is that it leads one toward the 'mini' aerosol types such as the Simoniz or the Styan Cub. But these are really too small to be relied upon for the kind of situation we may face on a boat. In my view they just don't hold enough extinguishant. On the other hand, it may be reasonable to have three or four of them around the boat to be used as 'side arms' to fight one's way to the bigger armament. In that way one can strike a reasonable balance between economy, effectiveness, and stowage space.

Cost, as I have implied, cannot be ignored. As may be deduced from other chapters in this book, one needs quite a large amount of safety gear aboard a boat and the cost quickly mounts up. Indeed, a shallow pocket is probably one of the most common causes of tragedy at sea, and I suspect that there are few among us amateur mariners who are as fully equipped with safety gear as we would wish. An extinguisher containing 4 lb or 5 lb weight of BCF for example will cost between £15 and £20 as I write (1976) and is not likely to become any cheaper as far as I can judge. Yet I think that a couple of that size would not be at all excessive for a boat of 25-feet length, assuming that she has an engine and the usual variety of inflammable fuels on board. £30 must be the *minimum* investment for fire-fighting gear in a 5- or 8-tonner, I think.

In addition I myself have several of the little aerosol units on board at a cost of about £2·00 each. But I could not rely on those alone – they are merely ancillaries.

One other decision has to be made, and that is in the choice of the actual brand of extinguisher. The problem here is that although BCF is coming into ever wider use in industry it is not currently found in retail shops except in the smallest sizes. If one wants a 3 lb, 5 lb, or 8 lb type for example, then one will probably have to go to the makers. There are several possible firms, but two who are set up to meet individual orders are Pyrene (Pyrene House, Sunbury-on-Thames, Middlesex) and Graviner (Poyle Mill Works, Poyle Lane, Colnbrook, Bucks). Both these companies make equipment of high quality, and their extinguishers are of the controllable discharge type.

That's to say you are not obliged to use the whole content of the bottle at one go.

Another well-established company, Minimax, has entered the small-boat field with a useful kit of parts which allows any boat-owner to arrange effective protection for the engine compartment and bilge space of his craft. The kit makes use of a 3 lb BCF extinguisher, of the controllable discharge type. Minimax's address is Manor Lane, Feltham, Middlesex.

The single-shot bottle is more likely to be found among the cheaper models because there is a manufacturing economy if a valve is omitted. The single-shot device needs a simple diaphragm, or thin metal closure that is pierced to release the vapour. It has the disadvantage that you cannot use just part of the contents but on the other hand the controllable type is more likely to develop a leak at the valve.

Fortunately leaks in even the cheapest aerosol models are quite rare, so long as they are well cared for. If the cannister is allowed to stand around in the wet and go rusty then it will not be long before the contents escape. Presumably the man who is sufficiently careless to treat his safety gear in that way will be the very one who does not take much trouble about checking his equipment from time to time. More thoughtful owners, on the other hand, can check the contents of their BCF extinguishers by 'feeling the weight' and listening to the 'sloshing' of the fluid.

7. If That Engine Stops . . .

As I have explained in Chapter One, when I first began work on this book it was not possible to get good, analytical records of boating accidents. But even at that time it was clear to anyone who took the trouble to read the reports in the *Lifeboat Journal*, the *Coastguard*, and wherever news of sea incidents were to be found, that propulsion failure was a very frequent reason for a Mayday call or a red flare.

Some years later, when the Royal National Lifeboat Institution very kindly put its computer records at my disposal, for the benefit of private boat owners in general, two facts became very clear:

In the first place it was confirmed that a high proportion of lifeboat sorties was being made in aid of boats with propulsion failure. Secondly, it also became clear that propulsion failure very rarely leads to fatalities.

That is the great difference between the two most common causes of a lifeboat call – *capsize* and *machinery failure*. While each of these types of incident clearly outnumbers any other (between them they account for more than half of the lifeboatmen's work) *capsize* is very clearly a killer, while *mechanical failure* is equally clearly not lethal.

Nevertheless, there are many good reasons why one should want to avoid propulsion failure, ranging from the risk to your own boat to the far more important matter of the nuisance, and even risk, to the volunteer lifeboatmen. Thus I have always gone out of my way to recommend to all motor boat owners that they should equip their boats with some stand-by means of propulsion.

Even without any experience of the sea it is obvious that to take yourself to sea relying on a single engine is to take a very big risk. If for any reason it ceases to run and the crew are unable to get it going again they will find themselves in an unenviable situation. For a start, it must not be supposed that the fellow who is a good amateur mechanic ashore and looks after his car engine will be able to make a good job of an emergency repair at sea. He is unlikely to have the facilities of his garage at home, even though he may have been wise enough to bring aboard a good supply of tools, spare parts and odds and ends that 'might come in handy'. Furthermore, it takes a clear head and a strong stomach to work on an engine while the boat is rolling and pitching, when tools won't stay still, and when a vital nut is most likely to roll down into that unreachable part of the bilge just beneath the engine bearers . . .

And while attempts are being made to get the engine running again, the boat herself may not be faring too well. Wind, or tide, or both may be carrying her into danger. Think, for example of the channel that leads out from Hurst Narrows to the Needles at the western end of the Isle of Wight – a scene that makes a lovely picture postcard subject on a fine day. But that piece of water which is so attractive to a fishing party in a motor boat abounds with dangers. On the one shore there are cliffs and rocky shoals, with some beaches in fairly well sheltered bays, it is true, but remember that one cannot choose one's point of impact with the land in a drifting boat . . .

On the other side of the channel is a steep-sided shingle bank which will mean almost certain destruction to any boat which should ground on it in heavy weather, while even a light-draft boat would fare badly in the turbulent breaking seas that form over the bank when wind and tide are strong.

At the seaward end of the Needles passage there are the rocks from which it takes its name plus an area of water with a reputation for roughness which makes many people take the alternative route whenever they can. And even at the inner end, just before you reach the sheltered waters of the Solent there is that shoal called The Trap at the tip of Hurst Point.

A fine catalogue of horrors to make your flesh creep, but there is still one more. The ships. They need the deep water of the channel of course, and the skipper of a small boat may very sensibly keep close to one edge or the other, so putting his craft nearer the natural dangers. But if the engine stops and there is no other means of propulsion the boat may swiftly be carried any which way, depending on the strengths and directions of wind and tide. Perhaps on to the Shingles, perhaps into the track of a ship, perhaps back into the Solent where you might eventually bump safely but ignominiously into the mud of Hampshire!

THE ANCHOR: SMALL-BOAT MARINER'S BEST FRIEND

But seamanlike readers will by this time have dropped their anchors, in imagination at least, and that of course is the sensible (and sometimes the only possible course of action. It cannot *always* be an effective answer because there are places where cliffs run straight down into deep water, too deep for the scope of cable carried aboard a pleasure craft. And there are places where the holding is bad, as it is on the Shingles aforementioned, where the bank is steep-sided and the round stones roll before the anchor. Nevertheless, in the case of engine failure (and I am assuming that there is no other means of

89

propulsion) which happens anywhere near land or shoal water it is good sense to lower the anchor on its full scope of cable, even though it may not yet find bottom. It will tend to steady the motion of the boat even while in deep water, and the anchor will have the earliest opportunity of getting a bite as soon as the boat does begin to enter the shallows. That will give you the best chance of coming to your anchor at a good distance off the shore.

Provided that the anchor will hold, that the cable is sound, and the seas are not of extraordinary severity, a motor boat may lie to her anchor for an indefinite period, depending on the supplies of food, the stamina of the crew, and the provisions they have made to protect themselves against exposure. Usually no great trial of endurance is required, because it does not take long for those aboard either to re-start the engine or to decide that they cannot do it. In the latter case a red flare brings out the lifeboat and that is the end of the matter, but to lie at anchor does give time for thought, for the tide to turn, for repairs to be made, for the sun to come up and put new heart into everybody, and above all it does keep the boat out of danger, even though her occupants may be wet, cold and bailing for their lives.

Truly, the anchor is the small-boat mariner's best friend but, let us attend here to the risks of engine failure.

RUNNING OUT OF FUEL

Clearly, all manner of things can go wrong with an engine, of which the simplest is that it runs out of fuel. This is evidently a far more serious matter at sea than it is by the roadside, yet it is quite a common cause of the lifeboat's being called out. I recall the time when a boat went missing on a delivery trip from Christchurch to the Channel Islands. The man who was making the delivery, as a job of work, set out with what he believed was just enough fuel for the passage. The boat was a small cabin craft, driven by a single outboard engine, and whether or not his calculation of 'just enough' was correct nobody will ever know because he disappeared somewhere, somehow on that passage and was never seen again. A sad tale, but one would have thought that even the least experienced of amateurs would make himself a generous allowance of fuel. An engine may consume more than you were led to expect. For example, on one boat I had an 8 h.p. Stuart Turner two-stroke whose consumption just about doubled if the throttle lever was moved from half-way to full open. But the speed of the boat, as is to be expected, increased by only about 10 or 15 per cent, so with the throttle full open her miles-per-gallon went down alarmingly. That was well understood, but I was caught out when the throttle developed a trick of opening itself – by vibration. I first became seriously aware of it when coming back from the West Country in a dead calm. We made a night passage across Lyme Bay and when I dipped the tank by day-light I was somewhat set back to see how little fuel was left. At first I suspected a leak (which is a very frightening suspicion to have when the fluid is petrol) but later I woke up to the fact that the throttle had slowly crept forward, bringing a slight increase in engine speed but a large increase in fuel flow. In short, my quite large reserve of fuel beyond what would have been strictly necessary for the passage to Weymouth had been used up before we had come abeam of Portland Bill. But the breeze came up with the sun, so we carried on under sail.

One may run out of fuel because of a leak, a miscalculation, or simply by forgetting to top up. In a sea-going boat I like to have two tanks, of which one has sufficient capacity for all normal work, while the other is the stand-by. Alternatively, where I have had only one tank I have always taken care to have plenty of spare fuel in proper, strongly-made cans, clearly marked and painted to distinguish them from any others on board. Incidentally, where there are two tanks I make it a practice to run from the stand-by at least once a year and try to use up at least three-quarters of its contents so that I can fill with fresh fuel before turning back to the main tank.

BLOCKAGE IN PIPES OR FILTERS

Apart from running out of fuel, the engine may be starved by a blockage in pipes or filters. This tends to happen at the most awkward times – in other words when the sea gets up a bit or when the boat is in the rougher water off a headland, because the movement stirs up sediment in the tank. The fuel pipe will have its inlet a slight distance above the bottom of the fuel tank, where there should also be a small depression or sink to act as a sludge trap. This normally keeps the fuel inlet clear of sediment, but when the fuel starts sloshing about in a seaway it is a different matter.

So – the answers are obvious. Once a year (or more if you like) it is worthwhile removing the drain plug, or the tap fitting from the bottom of the tank and drawing off a pint or so of the fuel in the hope that a good portion of the sediment will come with it. If the tank can be removed with reasonable ease – which is a rarity – then by all means remove it and clean it properly. The second answer is to keep the filters in the fuel line clean, and to know where they are so that you can get at them quickly if necessary.

In a water-cooled engine, as most marine inboards are, a blockage in the water line can also stop the engine, which may overheat and seize up. If the exhaust is water-cooled there may be trouble from that area too. Regrettably the chance of a blocked water intake is rather higher these days than it used to be because there are so many pieces of plastic sheeting floating around in the sea. Apart from knowing where the inlet strainer is, and how to clear it, it might also prove rewarding to devise a contingency plan for dealing with an external blockage due to a piece of plastic or cloth getting foul of the skin-fitting. One is unlikely to be able to do anything useful by poking about with a boathook – these intakes are nearly always quite inaccessible in that way. Nor can one assume that the sea will be calm enough to allow a good swimmer to go over the side to it. A more dependable line of thought might be to disconnect the engine inlet pipe and to connect to it a piece of hose that can be led straight over the side of the cockpit. That will probably be quite effective if the engine has a good water-pump, otherwise some priming may be necessary.

Fuel, water, lubricating oil are all essential to the running of an engine, but even when they are supplied there are many other things that can go wrong. It is at sea, under a grey sky and a mounting wind when white caps begin to blow from the tops of the waves, that one wishes there had been more time (or more will?) to give the engine the maintenance that it should have had. One merit in attending regularly to the maintenance of one's own engine is that one becomes more familiar with it, and so better able to cope if the need arises. Now this book is not intended as an engine maintenance manual, but the point must be made that safety at sea may depend on the presence of certain spare parts plus the tools to tackle the work. I have in mind such things as contact-breaker points, a spare capacitor, spare sparking plugs, and a spare coil for a petrol engine; spare injector nozzles or even a spare injector complete for a diesel engine; spare gaskets, fibre washers for fuel lines and so forth for any type of engine.

Some people may wish to carry a complete spare magneto –

if that particular component is frequently a source of trouble. Certainly a spare coil is essential in a spark-ignition boat, for when a coil packs up there is nothing to do but change it. Very extensive lists of spares may be made up by those who view the subject seriously, just as would be done by anybody setting off to cross the Kalahari Desert in a car. At sea, service stations and supplies of spare parts are just as remote as they are in the middle of the Kalahari.

DAMAGE TO THE PROPELLER

The single-engined boat is not only at the mercy of her engine, she may be crippled if her propeller is damaged, either by striking the bottom in shallow water, or more likely by striking some floating balk of timber or the like. Here again, both the twin-screw craft, and the craft with sail and power, have a second chance. Another hazard that affects propellers is the drifting fisherman's net, which is nowadays likely to be made of some lightweight synthetic material which floats, does not rot, and is strong. If one gets one of these around the prop then it is more than likely that it will not be cleared until the boat comes into harbour.

The same may be said of a single rope, such as may be attached to the floats marking lobster pots and other fishing gear whose exact character I do not know. These floats, usually marked with a flag which may or may not be easily visible, are found in large numbers around British coasts and are a real hazard. They are especially worrying when they are in constricted channels, such as those which often exist as a narrow bank of relatively smooth water between a race and a headland. The fishermen don't like to go out into the race either, so they lay their gear in the same narrow strip of water that the cruising boat wants to use. But this is just the place, between two

natural hazards, where one would prefer not to get involved
with a third, man-made snare.

Prevention is better than cure, and for my part I insist on an
arrangement of propeller and rudder which makes it difficult
for a rope or net to entwine itself around either.

But suppose that you do get something foul of prop or
rudder – there are several possible lines of action.

A single line which has been picked up by the propeller and
wound around the shaft a few times before bringing the engine
to a halt *may* be cleared by unwinding from the deck or cockpit.
If the end of the rope can be picked up with a boathook and
pulled firmly while the motor is turned over with the gear
engaged to turn the prop in reverse there is a chance that the

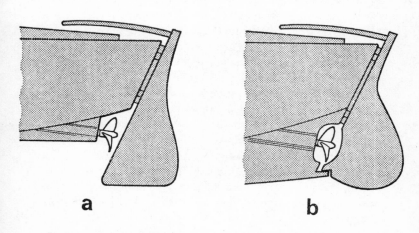

a   **b**

To tangle your dinghy painter around your prop-shaft is a bit of
a joke – but the RNLI is often called to a boat with a fouled
propeller or rudder. The arrangement at **a** seems to have been
designed to catch anything and everything. Myself, I prefer
something like **b**.

95

rope will come clear. In a petrol engine this is best done with the sparking plugs removed to relieve the compression so that the engine can be turned by hand. On a diesel the valve-lifter can be used if there is one fitted. If not you have a difficulty because you don't want to run the risk of starting the engine again – there's more than a chance that the rope will come almost free, then wind up again the other way.

In some boats it may be possible to see the tangle from the deck, and a sharp knife, or a hacksaw may be better, can be lashed to a boathook. But that is not often going to be possible, and it is much more likely that the job could be done from a dinghy. Nevertheless, serious thought must be given to the risk involved in trying to work close under the stern of a boat in a dinghy if there is any sea running. The same may be said of the last resort of putting a swimmer in the water – it is very easy to get a heavy bang on the head from the falling stern of a boat, even though one should have tried to make things easier by moving spare crew members and easily-shifted weights towards the bows so as to lift the stern a little.

If a swimmer does go over he must wear harness, keep a line attached to the boat, and be under the eye of an appointed guardian. It is best to attach the tools he will need to lengths of codline and to lower them over to him. He will then be able to 'put the saw down' so to speak if he suddenly needs both his hands to care for himself. It might look funny, but it would be sensible for him to wear some kind of head protection – even a woolly hat with some stuffing inside it would be better than nothing.

One thing which can be done, if ever you happen to have the propeller shaft out of the boat, is to slip a short length of loose sleeving over any exposed part of the shaft between deadwood and propeller. (Remember to allow for the fore and aft movement of some shafts which control variable pitch propellers.)

If that is done, a tightly wound rope will be tight only around the loose sleeving, and not around the shaft as normally happens. Thus the prop may still be free to turn, and the rope should be easier to free.

Indirectly related to safety, but we once went about for several days with a woolly hat wrapped around the prop, wondering why the engine revs were down and why speed was down even more. The same can happen with a piece of plastic fertiliser bag, or even with thick seaweed. Often a burst in reverse will clear it – otherwise one has to proceed in the same way as for a tangled rope.

A SECOND SOURCE OF PROPULSION

But whether it's a rope round the prop, water in the fuel, a failed ignition coil or any other cause that brings your engine to a stop, any skipper must feel very much happier if he has some alternative means of propulsion that can be brought into use. I am still regularly surprised by the number of people who put to sea relying on the power of just one engine – relying upon the continued working of an assembly of parts and components any one of which may by its failure bring the whole expedition to a halt. And it is not only a matter of safety – it can be downright embarrassing to come to a halt even in conditions of perfect safety. We once 'rescued' a party in a powerful ski-boat which was hanging on to a mooring in a sheltered creek not more than half a mile from the quay where they had parked their car. That was as far as they had been able to get before their engine came to a stop (as it later turned out, with oiled-up plugs, but they had no spanner). As they had no anchor and no other means of propulsion, the best they could do was to grab a mooring buoy as they drifted past. When we found them they were on the edge of the mud, for the tide had ebbed, and, tired of their enforced and inactive wait, one of their number was some hundreds of yards away, floundering up to his waist in mud, trying to get ashore for help. All very silly and trivial, but it does illustrate the point. In a quieter creek, and in slightly deeper water, they might have had to stay there the whole night before some other boat happened to pass.

SECOND INBOARD ENGINE

With two engines, of course, the picture becomes very different. The chance of having an engine failure is doubled, but the chance of complete power loss is very much reduced – provided that each engine has its own independent supply of fuel and cooling water. But a full twin-engined installation is expensive, like so many of the things one needs for safety in a boat.

EMERGENCY OUTBOARD ENGINE

If the boat has a tender and if the tender has an outboard motor, then it may be considered as a reserve against emergency. In a calm and with not much headwind, even a 3 or 4 h.p. outboard will bring a 30-foot boat back to harbour – so long as there is sufficient fuel. But in such a case the wise skipper will make the best use he can of wind and tide because he simply will not have the power to fight against them. Nevertheless the motive power may enable him to get to some point of refuge downwind, even if it is not precisely the place you would have chosen in happier circumstances.

If one is to rely upon the tender's outboard as a second source of power then it will be best to try and work out (in advance, of course) some way in which the motor can be attached directly to the bigger boat herself. It may be difficult to find a place for it on the transom, and even if it is physically possible, one has to think of the problem that comes when the boat starts pitching – the motor may be under the water at one moment, and high in the air with screw screaming round at the next. It will not last long. There may be better conditions for the outboard if it can be mounted on the side of the boat – perhaps alongside the cockpit. It may be necessary to devise special brackets, but as a makeshift a board lashed right across the cockpit with one end overhanging by about 12 to 18 inches can make a basis for an outboard mounting.

Towing the boat from an outboard-powered dinghy may prove satisfactory, though if there is any sea a long, heavy line (perhaps specially weighted) may be required to absorb the snatch. The load on the dinghy will be very severe, and unless a high level of seamanship is exercised there is danger that she will be swamped. With most boats and most dinghies a better solution will be to 'moor' the dinghy alongside her parent craft, with breast-ropes and springs, and fenders between. With her outboard running, and nobody aboard her, the dinghy will do a better job like that.

MAKESHIFT SAILING RIG

There are many permutations, of course, in the case of engine failure, so one cannot lay down any rules. A small motor cruiser with a failed engine could blow down wind, or even at 45 degrees to left or right of the direct downwind course, if the owner were able to set some sort of sail, and if she had a rudder. By no means every power craft can be made to carry sail, and there is not much hope for the planing and high-speed types. But a displacement-type of motor cruiser can usually be rigged to make reasonably good use of a modest

99

amount of sail area, which may also be used to save fuel and yield a little peace and quiet on ordinary passages – when the wind is favourable. Just as virtually all sailing cruisers now carry a powerful 'auxiliary' engine, so I believe that more motor cruisers will come to be rigged as motor-sailers, so providing one answer to the problem posed by going to sea in a single-engined craft.

The sail may be a bed-sheet, or a cockpit cover, or almost anything, and the mast might be a boathook or an oar. But these makeshift contrivances will be difficult to rig if there is any movement on the sea, so the best policy is to experiment at leisure and preferably to make some bits and pieces of gear which can be assembled in a pre-planned scheme.

I said 'if she has a rudder', because many outboard-powered boats do not have a rudder. In that case an oar over the stern might have to do the job, though it is not always as easy as it sounds unless some preparation has been made. Ideally a boat designed and built without a rudder (i.e. depending on the turning of the propeller from side to side for steering) should have special provision made for shipping a jury rudder. But that is Utopia. In a real world the owner himself will have to devise something, and if he leaves it until the day when he's in trouble he will find himself trying the old business of screwing a locker-door on to a floorboard, or something equally impractical.

OARS

In small motor boats and sailing dinghies there is just the same need for alternative means of propulsion, and one or more pairs of oars will provide one answer. A paddle, on the other hand, is not worth the space it takes up. It is true that oars occupy a lot of space, but they are effective if rowlocks can be shipped and if the oarsman has a good working position. Not so very long ago, before internal combustion engines were generally available, cruising boats up to 5 tons displacement were propelled by the oar in time of calm. (In France they are still.) Either that, or they stayed where they were, at anchor, or drifted wheresoever the current might take them. So don't spurn a pair of oars – even two pairs if there is space enough for two occupants of the boat to row simultaneously, because really remarkable progress can be made with two people pulling.

For real security on cruising boats the real answer is to have a properly worked-out arrangement, whether it be a modest sailing rig, a second inboard engine, or a properly-fitted bracket to carry an outboard chosen for the purpose.

POISONOUS EXHAUST GASES

One further danger relating to the engine deserves a mention – the leaky exhaust. Petrol engine exhaust gases contain a high proportion of carbon monoxide, which everybody knows is a lethally poisonous gas. In the open air the exhaust from a motor car rarely has any harmful effect, but there is much more risk in the confined space of a boat. In boats exhaust pipes often run in confined spaces which communicate directly with the cabin, and there are a good many recorded cases of people being overcome by exhaust fumes.

The danger is made more real by the corrosion to which metal fittings on boats are subject. Furthermore, owners sometimes allow their exhaust pipes to become choked by carbon deposits ...

It should not be necessary to say more. If one is aware of the danger it is possible to keep a sharp look-out for the chance of a leak.

8. The Prudent Sailor

I will not join the many writers who have made up for their own lack of experience of the heaviest sea conditions by trying to recommend any one of the several possible heavy-weather procedures, or rehearse the arguments for and against sea anchors (the balance of opinion is heavily against) and over rival methods of heaving to. I have never experienced anything above Force 8 (and that not for long), and I hope to end my days in the same happy ignorance. In fact, the sort of average boat-owner whom I have in mind as I write this book is likely to avoid the heaviest weather too, by listening to the shipping forecasts, and never taking any chances.

As I have implied in an earlier chapter, stress of weather is one of the rarer causes of injury and tragedy among small craft and their crews. But it is a subject which naturally attracts a great deal of attention, and one which occupies a place of importance in many of the books one reads about ocean voyages in cruising boats. But the fact is that these accounts of long-distance voyages throw the whole matter out of perspective. I think it very important for the ordinary owner of a small sea-going boat to recognise the fundamental difference between ocean voyaging and coastal cruising.

The ocean-voyaging man will be at sea for months or weeks. Thus he must take the weather as it comes, and the best he can do is to plan his passages outside the known hurricane seasons. The weekend and holidays cruising man, on the other hand, is usually at sea for less than twelve hours, and only rarely for more than twenty-four hours. It is therefore much easier for him to avoid bad conditions by leaning on the professional forecasters. He may also supplement their judgement by his own deductions based upon observation of the barometer, thermometer and other signs. I have little faith in such amateur methods myself, and will leave them to those who propound them enthusiastically in their own books or articles.

The fact remains, that for most of us, the principal aim is to avoid heavy weather, a thing which the ocean-voyaging skipper has little chance of doing. The only category of non-professional seaman who must expect to face bad weather, then, is the ocean-racing chap. In Adlard Coles' book *Heavy Weather Sailing* there are hair-raising accounts of the things that happened to superb ocean-racing yachts manned by strong crews. Some of those gales and storms I still remember, and I also recall that I was safely in port at the time, along with many other family cruisers. That was the prudent, seamanlike thing to do. Indeed, I don't think that there can be many cruising families who need to be told . . . anyone who has sailed in a Force 6 wind, let alone 7, will not wish to find himself out in Force 8.

People who want to go in for long-distance voyaging, or ocean racing, will study seamanship at a level far beyond anything that I could offer. My concern is with the far greater numbers of ordinary people who want to do a little 'pleasure boating'. They need not feel ashamed if prudence borders on timidity; I know one small-boat skipper who for the past twenty years or more has kept clear of trouble by taking great care not to expose himself or his boat to the least chance of bad weather. He seems to me to get just as much pleasure from his boating as anybody else – and as a former professional seaman he knows what he's about.

WIND FORCE AND REEFING

On the other hand you get the reckless sort, and also those who are not so much reckless as deluded into thinking a spirit of 'press on regardless' is the sign of the true seaman. By way of a specific example, reefing and the judgement of when or whether to reef is a clear case where prudence and bravado have their exponents. It has often been said, and it is still true, that a boat when cruising should be comfortable in gusts and slightly under-canvassed for the rest of the time: but that in racing a boat should be over-canvassed in the puffs because she would be carrying full sail the rest of the time. There is all the difference between one's conduct when racing and when cruising. Reefing is hardly acceptable in a race, but it would be a great mistake to go cruising in a racing frame of mind, especially in an open boat or in the typical family-crewed cruiser.

In contrast to the open boat, the decked and cabined cruiser is not going to be put into immediate danger by carrying too much sail, but she will tire her crew, become difficult to manage, and may ultimately overload her gear – perhaps suffer serious damage such as the loss of a mast.

A great deal of nonsense is talked about reefing, especially of the kind, 'Oh, we never reef until Force 5 . . .' The speaker may be telling the truth, but if he understood the matter a little better he would keep his mouth shut – or at least he would utter the same words in tones of regret rather than pride. For if he really does not reef until Force 5 his boat must be grossly under-canvassed in Force 3 and 2, when sailing should be such a pleasure. In Force 3 the wind pressure on each square foot of sail is *five times* smaller than it is in Force 5, so it is obvious that the same sail area will not do for both conditions.

The Beaufort scale is a measure of wind *speed*, and it is rather misleading that it uses the word 'force'. 'Force' should really imply *push* or *thrust*, which varies in proportion to the square of the wind speed. In other words, if the wind speed is doubled the force on each square foot of sail increases four-fold. Perhaps the following table will be helpful: it is a rough guide to the relative push one would get from a given area of sail at different wind speeds.

Wind speed range knots	Beaufort 'force' number	Relative force exerted on unit sail area (approx.)
Less than 1	0	0
1–3	1	1
4–6	2	5
7–10	3	18
11–16	4	45
17–21	5	90
22–27	6	150
28–33	7	230
34–40	8	390
41–47	9	485

Ignoring the frightening figures towards the end of the table (they represent circumstances which I hope to avoid by careful attention to weather trends) it is quite obvious why large changes in sail area are needed to adjust to changes in wind speed. For the same thrust the sail area in Force 4, say, needs to be seven or eight times smaller than it would be in Force 2. In practice that is not achieved, nor is the problem quite so simple as that because there are other factors involved, but the underlying fact remains the same – it is the fundamentally under-canvassed boat which is reefed late.

But quite apart from that, there is good sense in reefing too early rather than too late. The job can become difficult when the boat is overpressed and the sea has become rough. Furthermore, many boats will go faster if they are relieved of a pressure of canvas which makes the hull heel over to an angle where the water drag becomes excessive, and where the degree of weather helm imposes additional drag in the water as well as an almost intolerable drag on the helmsman's arm.

Reefing usually depends on the wind conditions as they are at present, though the sensible seaman may well reef *now* because he expects bad conditions *later*. It is, for example, a good idea to reef while in harbour even though it may not seem strictly necessary in the light of conditions outside, if one thinks that before long it might become necessary. Better by far to do the job (and do it better) while the boat is at rest than in a tumbling sea where risks are always present.

THE WEATHER FORECAST

Or the real question may be whether to go out at all, reefed or not, and in taking that decision the best guide is without doubt the forecast provided by the Meteorological Office. Amateur forecasting gives some people a great deal of pleasure, but the information available to them is very limited and in no way comparable to that which the Met. Officer has at hand. And there is also the slight matter of his training and skill . . .

So a radio receiver is a primary safety instrument for anyone who plans to take a boat to sea – not only for the warnings of gales and strong winds, but also for forecasts of fog and mist which can be a real danger to craft close to the shore or in the shipping lanes.

Personally, I find it absolutely necessary to write down the forecast for the shipping area or areas in which I am interested, and usually one is interested in at least two – that's to say the area in which you actually are, and the area from which the weather is coming. If I don't write it down I find that five seconds later I have forgotten what the man said – which is natural enough because the memory is overlaid by his subsequent forecasts for successive regions.

It is useful to listen to all types of forecast when one really needs to know what the weather trend is, and that includes the land area forecasts with which most people are familiar. I will not list all the times here because changes are made as the years go by, and the full information can be had from *Reed's Almanac*, or from a copy of the *Radio Times*. The latter source is much cheaper for the owner of an open boat who may consider *Reed's* an unjustifiable expense for his purposes, though I think that any boat owner can find his money's worth in that mine of information.

The shipping forecasts by the BBC are broadcast on 1500 metres (200 kHz) which is on the 'long wave' band. Some cheap transistor receivers omit the long waves, and are therefore a bad buy for a mariner. The same frequency is used for gale warnings which are inserted into the BBC's normal programmes between shipping forecasts when necessary.

Not to be found in the *Radio Times* are details of the forecasts from Post Office Coastal Radio Stations, which broadcast on short waves in the band from 1600 to 3800 kHz. These stations give navigational warnings, and shipping forecasts for areas in their vicinity, and it so happens that their weather forecasts fall nicely into certain gaps between the BBC's transmissions. There are more than a dozen of these stations around the shores of the United Kingdom, and their transmission times and frequencies are in *Reed's*, of course.

Apart from the broadcast forecasts it is always possible to make a direct inquiry by telephone. There are the recorded forecasts for local areas, for which you simply dial the number shown in the directory, but in major cities there is a Weather Centre which gives a more personal service. Weather Centres are run by the Met. Office. Some of them are situated at aerodromes, but in each case you have the opportunity to put direct questions to a trained forecaster. The full list, with telephone numbers, is in *Reed's Almanac* of course, and there is also the very useful pamphlet published by HMSO called *Your Weather Service*.

If in doubt one can always ring the nearest aerodrome, military or civil, and ask for the 'Forecast Office'. It will be rare indeed that help is not given willingly. Although personalities must play their part, and some forecasters are naturally more forthcoming than others, the personal contact can be very reassuring, and I have been surprised to find how often the chap at the other end of the line understands the problems of the small-boat skipper. Indeed, I am sure that there must be a high proportion of boat owners among forecasters.

It is obvious that there are plenty of ways of getting information about the trend of the weather. Day boats can get the information before they set out, and cabin boats can carry a small transistor radio, though it is important to be sure that the set will receive the 200 kiloHertz (i.e. 1500 metres) transmission.

But radio is not the only thing. For local gales harbours and signal stations still fly the black cone – point up for a northerly gale, point down for a southerly gale. *And* people still go on launching small boats within sight of a black cone and having to be rescued by the RNLI! Anyone who is a beginner may be excused for not knowing what the black cone means: but it is harder to excuse the chap who does not try to learn. If he is inexperienced then surely he should ask the harbourmaster or some other responsible person for an opinion on the likely weather before he commits himself to the sea. Even less understandable is the person who knows that a gale is forecast and yet ignores it. A gale warning implies that a wind of Force 8 or more is expected, and such a wind will make conditions *very* difficult for any small craft. Even Force 6 is enough for most owners of average-sized yachts, and as I have tried to show, there is a world of difference between the actual power of a Force 6 and a Force 8.

A point which is not always understood is that the terms used in broadcast warnings have a precise meaning. When a gale is said to be *imminent* it is expected to arrive in the area within 6 hours. *Soon* means some time between 6 and 12 hours, and *later* means beyond 12 hours.

My wife and I had to bring our boat back from Devon to the Solent some years ago, and we were dogged by gales. We lay all day in the deep and sheltered cleft of the River Dart (and even there the wind was howling through our rigging) and when we turned in that night the forecast was for more gales. But in that strange way that happens when one is afloat, I awoke at about five the next morning aware that there had been a change. I went ashore and rang the forecast office in Plymouth where a young woman confirmed that the wind had eased off but that gales would be back later. The 0640 shipping forecast also offered south-west winds of Force 4 or 5 to be followed by a south-westerly gale 'later'.

Being naturally cautious I made preparations to depart, but went ashore again for one more telephone call to the Met. man in Plymouth. The chap I spoke to this time was willing to bet his shirt that we would be free from the gale certainly until two o'clock in the afternoon and almost certainly till five or six in the evening. That would at least see us as far as Weymouth, so off we went for a fast sail in the imposing seas which had been built up by the previous days' gales. When the 1355 Shipping Forecast came on the air we were somewhere in the region of Portland Bill, and the gale was now forecast as 'soon' and from the south. We settled for Weymouth even though the expected timing should have allowed us to get on to Poole, say.

In fact that gale never came – the next day we had light winds and fog. Indeed, the gale that is forecast and does not arrive is a pleasantly familiar one, and far to be preferred to the gale that arrives without warning! Fortunately the second kind is as rare as the first is common. But the central point, as I see it, is that it is far better to be on the safe side. If in doubt, don't go out. Or if you do go out for a look, and don't like what you find, never feel that you will lose face if you turn back. Anyone with knowledge will recognise your good sense – not that its anybody else's business anyway.

STUDYING THE COURSE

It is often said to be a good thing to go out and have a look, because if one lies long enough in a sheltered harbour a sort of inertia or mental paralysis can set in. 'It may not be nearly so bad outside as you imagine', is how the argument runs, and there is a lot of truth in it. But the difficult problem is not the state of the sea outside your present harbour, it is the future state of the sea over the bar of the harbour you hope to enter some hours hence. Or it may be a matter of the sea conditions where a race forms off some headland that you must pass on your way . . . or the visibility some hours hence, at some crucial point on the route. For example, there are some narrow channels frequented by large ships which offer no possibility of protection by creeping into the shallows because their shores are dangerous with rocks and shoals. That is the sort of place I dread to enter in bad visibility.

Some experience, of course, is needed to appreciate even the existence of places where there will be overfalls, tide rips and other awkward sea states. Many headlands continue as shallow ridges beneath the water, and as the tidal stream is forced to accelerate around the headland it meets these shoals at increased speed, so forming the overfalls and standing waves that can be seen in miniature where a fast stream runs over a rocky bottom. At sea a race is usually something to be avoided at all costs, especially a big and powerful one like that off the tip of Portland Bill. Hilaire Belloc had much to say of Portland race (he had much to say of many things) and he accorded it a great respect. 'It lumps, hops, seethes and bubbles, just like water boiling over the fire, but the jumps are here in feet and the drops are in tons. There is no set of the sea in Portland Race; no run and sway; no regular assault. It is a chaos of pyramidical waters leaping up suddenly without calculation, or rule of advance.'

And much, much more he had to say, all of it enough to instil into any sailor a mortal fear of that famous race. But there are other, less lively races which are nevertheless enough to cause trouble for smaller boats, and especially for open ones. And because these are not so famous they may not come to the notice of the too casual sailor. The answer to that is not to be casual about the sea. There are pilot books which tell one how to circumvent these dangers. Charts bear warnings too, and some (Stanfords) have extensive pilotage information on their backs.

Careful study of chart and pilot before sailing is an essential safety technique. They will reveal the positions of wrecks, rocks, races, shoals and the like. They will warn about bars at harbour mouths, those shallow areas where the sea breaks right across your line of entry, especially when the ebb tide is pouring out of the harbour and into an onshore wind. Harbour is an attractive place when the sea is rough, the sky is grey, and morale is low, but the approach to it may be the most dangerous part of the whole passage. Indeed any approach to the land implies risks – first because the shallowing water and faster-running tidal streams can generate breaking seas, and second because there is something solid to hit, whether it be rocks or sand.

RIDING OUT OR RUNNING FOR SHELTER

The *really* prudent sailor will turn his ship towards the open sea when conditions become severe, because away from shore the seas come more regularly, are not so steep and rarely break. But few of us have the strength of will to take that course, and if we have been careful and fortunate in collecting the weather prognostications we may live a whole sailing life and never face the dilemma of deciding whether conditions are severe enough to necessitate an estrangement from the land. I suspect that on most occasions, most of us would tend to ignore the advice that was tendered over a hundred years ago by Richard McMullen and repeated in almost every cruising manual ever since. Contrary to the doctrine, we should most of us tend to turn landward in search of shelter.

And in point of fact I am not so sure that that is always such a bad decision, for on most such occasions we should be running for a haven in conditions which are less severe than McMullen had in mind when he said 'I am convinced that unless a small vessel, especially an open one, can be got into harbour before the sea becomes very heavy, there is more safety in keeping to the deep water and in not attempting to approach the land at all; where, owing to shallow water or currents, the sea will generally be far more dangerous.'

He went on to say that in the majority of cases when fishing boats were lost they were 'swallowed up near the shore, and often at the harbour's mouth'. He is generally credited with having been the first explicitly to make the point that small craft were safer well offshore in heavy weather. But the question remains, how heavy is heavy? With modern forecasting and the ability to make haste that is conferred by the auxiliary engine, our chances of being caught out are reduced. Furthermore, there is justification in trying to get into harbour when we have to share our waters with heavy commercial vessels which pose a serious threat of destruction to small craft. Many people fear big ships more than they fear big seas, and the only real defence against being run down is to keep a very sharp look-out. Yet to keep a good watch from a small boat in the sort of weather which would suggest standing off the land is an almost impossible task. The crew may be just a middle-aged man and woman, both of whom will soon be very tired, and perhaps seasick too. Their eyes will be smarting with salt, and visibility will be severely limited by flying spume or by rain.

In such conditions the crew will become accident-prone, and their weakness may prove a greater danger than the shallow and turbulent inshore waters. In short the *ship* may be better off at sea (though her manoeuvrability may be very limited) but the *crew* will very likely be worse off. The final judgement can be made only by the man on the spot, and will depend very much on the choices that are actually open.

In balancing the facts the prudent skipper will always have in mind the best haven to run for in any likely conditions. My own home port, Chichester, has a shallow entrance with a bar on which seas break from time to time. But 3 miles west there is a harbour with a deeper and safer entrance channel, and further west still there is the Solent with a wide selection of harbours, providing a safe entrance somewhere or other, no matter what quarter the weather is in. In that particular area we should have to be very imprudent to get ourselves into trouble by seeking a comfortable anchorage in heavy weather. Other parts of the coast are not so well arranged, of course, but whether one is in home waters or far away, it is always important to have in the back of one's mind the possibilities of shelter in case the weather comes up from an unexpected quarter.

Shelter does not necessarily imply entering a harbour – there are many naturally protected roadsteads which were much better known in the past than they are today, for the engine-less coasters and fishermen of those days had often to anchor in wait for a fair wind – or for a foul wind to blow over. The first cruising men used to share these roadsteads with commercial craft, for they too had no engines and if they could not get forward under sail they were obliged to use their anchors to avoid going backwards ... The fact that modern cruising people make so little use of such roadsteads as the Downs and Small Downs (east of Dover) or the sheltered bays under the lee of the Isle of Wight, or that behind the Start peninsula, shows very well how different are our circumstances nowadays. If the wind does not serve we proceed under engine. And it is also the 'iron topsail' that makes it easy for us to *enter* harbour and get safely into a berth, a thing that was not at all easy under sail alone with an offshore wind.

But the land is still there, and it will still provide shelter, provided that the boat has good anchors and cables, and a skipper who has cultivated his knowledge of seamanship and knows how to make best use of them. Lying in such a shelter in heavy weather will not be idyllic. The boat will roll and snatch, but she will be safe, and the crew will be able to conserve their strength. No longer obliged to keep a good look-out they must still be watchful, alert to any possible shift in the weather which might either make their position untenable, or more hopefully give them a chance to make progress towards a better haven.

BAD VISIBILITY

Although storms at sea cause a great deal of misgiving, it would not seem that they are the cause of a high proportion of the troubles that small craft get into. Probably, bad visibility is a more serious threat, and a good reason why any boat which is to go more than a mile off the shore should carry a compass, a chart, and a leadline. Many people have not experienced the speed with which a sea mist can roll in and blot out the scene. At one moment you are basting under a hot sun, rubbing oil into back and arms, and ten minutes later you will be shivering in a cold white mist and unable to see more than a hundred yards in any direction. That may not happen very often – but once could be enough. A more frequent cause of bad visibility is heavy rain – something which people do not appreciate until they have been at sea with low cloud and a severe rainstorm.

THE CREW'S MORALE A VITAL CONSIDERATION

Not only is the actual visibility reduced, one's morale falls too. Many brave and experienced seamen, chaps who have sailed round the world and across oceans, have admitted that their spirits fall when the sky turns grey and gives the sea a cold, threatening look. A stiff breeze and white horses make a jolly sight when the sun is shining, but the same sea and wind force take on a very unkind expression under ten-tenths cloud.

And as the sea gets rougher people may be numbed by a mental lassitude, a kind of inertia in which any constructive effort seems too difficult. It becomes too much of an effort to consult the chart, to reef a sail, or indeed to do more than hunch numbly at the tiller, hoping that it will soon be over. This mood is in fact one of the real dangers of seagoing, and we must try to recognise its onset and master it. There is no call for shame – it is something that is widely shared and it need not be dangerous as long as we have the sense to prepare our minds long in advance, so that we remember that a conscious effort must be made when lassitude invades the spirit.

If actual seasickness afflicts you, then the will to work may be completely undermined. It is no exaggeration to say that people suffering from seasickness may not have the will to save themselves by putting on lifejackets or getting into a liferaft – should it come to such a situation. It requires a supreme effort of will to continue working, and to work effectively, when you are feeling really seasick. For that reason it is an important safety principle to see that members of the crew who suffer from this unpleasant and serious malady are provided with the necessary pills in good time. The choice of drugs is mainly a matter for each individual, for different drugs are effective for different people. But extensive tests made by the Ministry of Defence show that compounds of hyoscine are most effective for the greatest number of people. Many proprietary travel sickness pills contain hyoscine hydrobromide, hyosciamine or other combinations of this drug. An advantage of hyoscine is that it does not cause drowsiness as some others do, though it does dry the mouth and may make the head feel hot. Drink plenty of water when taking hyoscine.

To be alert, free from seasickness, and warm and dry – all these are good safety points. They will reduce the chance of a foolish error which leads to worse trouble, and they will make the crew better able to cope with any unavoidable difficulties that do arise. If you are feeling as comfortable and fit as is possible in the circumstances (and the truth is that circum-

stances at sea in a small boat can be utterly miserable at times)
then there is less chance that you will fire your distress signals
when it is not strictly necessary. It is not at all uncommon for
people to fire red flares from boats which, as the experts leaning
on the bar are quick to comment, could easily have been
brought to safety under their own power. In such cases it is
evident that although some other person 'could easily have
brought her in', the job was beyond the abilities of that particular skipper and crew at that time. Their morale was already
so low that they were past effective action: their minds had
reached that numbed state of resignation when mental effort
becomes impossible. The subsequent censure of onlookers
does not alter the fact that that particular crew *was* in real
danger, even though it was not so much from the sea as from
their own limitations.

At times like that much depends on the skipper, and on his
power to sustain the spirits of the rest of the crew – which in
the context of this book will usually mean his own family. He
has to bear the burden of making the decisions, of seeing them
carried out, of facing the fact that lives will depend on his
judgement and ability, *and* of doing all those things with a
brave face. Blustering, shortness of temper, sarcasm and other
such displays of emotion undermine confidence. Sensible,
steady behaviour, and a cheerfulness which is appropriate to
the moment and not incongruously excessive, are what is
needed.

But prudence, of course, implies that one avoids getting
oneself and one's crew into situations beyond their capabilities.
What is perfectly reasonable for one man is not acceptable for
another, and that means that no skipper should be tempted to
take a course of action just because somebody else is doing it.
If somebody else is pushing out into the night when Force 6
is forecast it may be that he is either very competent or very

foolish. If you feel that Force 3 is the limit for your boat and your team it is a matter for you alone. Above all, no skipper should ever force his family out into weather that will make any one of them frightened or unhappy. A strained emotional atmosphere in a family boat is the prelude to errors of judgement – and in any case we are all supposed to be doing it for pleasure, are we not?

Having done one's best not to take on conditions that are too much for the particular crew involved, it is also necessary to attend to all those things which will keep the crew working efficiently – and that means adequate food, adequate clothing and adequate rest. Now although I talk about the 'skipper' who is usually also father, a family boat is a joint husband and wife affair. Food and clothing are likely to be in a wife's province, and she will certainly be able to improvise what is necessary and appropriate. The average family will not normally make very long sea passages, twelve or sixteen hours may rarely be exceeded, and periods of less than eight hours will be more normal. Therefore, a good hot meal at the start and finish of the trip will need to be supplemented only by snacks and hot drinks (or cold ones if you are really lucky with the weather) while under way. Snacks are so varied that there is little to be said – it may be fruit cake, biscuits, chocolate, sandwiches, pies, cold sausages, or anything that people fancy. Dried apricots, sultanas, and the sweet soft prunes suit my own palate, though I'll always join in and take my share of anything that's going . . .

Hot drinks can be a little more difficult. If neither adult member of the crew has the stomach to go below and work at the cooker (a very common weakness) then the obvious thing is to fill vacuum flasks. Otherwise one has all the usual range of hot drinks and soups at one's disposal. Much depends on the sea state, whether it be calm or rough, but if the latter then the greatest care must be taken with hot liquids. The 'cook' will be well advised to wear oilskins as protection.

In some respects a family group may be worse off than the single-hander because father's attention and morale may be undermined if he has sick, cold or frightened people on his conscience. If he can remain detached from such considerations it will be a different matter again. Nevertheless, most families plan their cruises in short port-to-port hops in the hours of daylight. That is a procedure which fits in with the natural rhythm of sleeping and waking, and so avoids any special attention to the problem of rest. Where the crew is physically stronger, as when there are four or five hearty young men, or where night passages must be made, then the skipper (backed up by mother) must ensure that people get their proper rest.

If all are allowed to stay on deck all the time, each claiming that he is a superhuman who needs no rest, there is a fair chance that when the need does arise nobody will be capable of meeting it. And chief among those who need rest is the skipper himself, of course. As he is the key figure, he must first arrange his rest period for a time when the going is easy, and then fit the watches of other crew members into a suitable pattern.

There are many variables in this business of the human factor, but the rule must always be not to overtax the crew as a whole. One can never predict when some kind of 'emergency' may arise, and it is important that the crew should always be in a fit state to cope. It is also worth remembering that everyone takes a day or two to get his 'sea-legs' and to settle down to life afloat. Therefore, I don't think it wise to plan anything ambitious for the first day of a cruise: that is a time for a shakedown, for people to get their minds and bodies in tune with the life on board.

THE PRUDENT SKIPPER DOES HIS
HOMEWORK FIRST

This first twenty-four hours or so is a period in which mother can check stores, and plan sustenance for the morrow, while father checks the boat's gear and prepares his passage plan. This is not intended to be a treatise on seamanship, but the safety of the ship is obviously going to depend in large measure on the skipper's pilotage, and that will be made the more certain if he has made good notes of such things as the set of tides, notable buoys, light characteristics, special hazards and the like before setting off. He will in addition, being the prudent seaman that he is, have considered alternative harbours of refuge, and what he might do IF . . . if the weather blows up and he wants to run back, if the visibility should close in, if tomorrow's forecast is not quite what he would have hoped, and so forth.

9. The Wrong Kind
of Dinghy

'Hello, is that the editor – I wonder if you could give me some advice about buying a sailing dinghy?'

The woman on the telephone, I thought, must be a young mother. I could hear baby noises in the background. She told me that she and her husband had been to see a plywood sailing dinghy, and she wanted to know if plywood was a suitable material for boats, and would it last, and did I think her husband could repair it, and was the price right, and . . .

Well, one does the best one can. But the thing I really wanted to know was what sort of dinghy it was. That point, it seemed, had not arisen during their Sunday afternoon at the boatyard, but she would ring them and ask, then ring me again. Ten minutes later she told me it was an *Enterprise*, and now it was my turn to put a few questions. Had they any experience? – not much? Were they going to take the infant I could hear? 'Oh yes, it's just me and my husband and the baby, and my friend and her husband.'

'Has your friend got a baby too?' (I wondered if I was beginning to sound a little sarcastic by now.)

'Oh no. But she is expecting one,' replied my female friend, sounding as if she expected me to take as much joy in the good news as she herself obviously did.

Then began a long conversation which almost turned into a

121

dispute as I tried to explain to her why an *Enterprise* was not a type of boat suited to their needs. I explained that she is a racing boat. 'But *we* won't race', she said in the tones of a young man who thinks he may have a motor bike if he promises never to go above 40 m.p.h. I persevered and finally persuaded her (I think) that she and her husband should go to a dinghy exhibition that was shortly to be held in London, so that they could see the various types available and discuss them with people of experience.

It is in fact not always easy to explain to people that there are two very different kinds of sailing dinghy, not to mention those that stand half-way, so to speak. A long time ago there was really only one type of sailing dinghy (or so it seems in retrospect), a type developed from the sea-going boats of the fishermen and so well able to take care of their crews. Working boats had to be able to do that because the crew would be busy with their lines and nets, and sometimes they would burden their boats with very heavy loads. Such sailing boats were not fast in the modern sense because they did not have the ability to plane.

It was Uffa Fox who changed it all in 1927, and especially 1928, when *Avenger*, his 14-foot *International* swept all the opposition before her. Uffa had applied ideas from the hydro-planes of the day to sailing boats, and by giving his dinghies a broad flat run aft was able to make them skim or plane over the surface of the water in a fresh breeze. Perhaps 'skim' is not quite the right word, but planing in dinghies is too complex a matter to analyse here. But planing, when the boat accelerates quite remarkably, is not achieved only by hull form, it also requires a high power-to-weight ratio – in other words a large sail area in proportion to the size and weight of the boat. That in turn means that the crew must sit with *their* weight out to windward so as to hold the boat upright.

All this provides great fun, of course, and also involves a good deal of agility and quick responses on the part of the crew. Nowadays it is usually forgotten that the 14s as Uffa used to sail them had a heavy bronze centreplate with a weight of about 120 lb, and that made them a very different boat from the modern 14 with her wooden centreboard. When a boat is on a more or less level keel a heavy drop-plate has little or no righting effect. On the other hand the weight of the crew to one side or the other exerts large leverage which can be used to good effect. But when a boat is heeled over on to her beam-ends the weight of the crew on one gunwale has no righting influence because it is now above the centre of buoyancy. This is just when a heavy keel, sticking out horizontally, has its greatest leverage and does most to right the boat. In later years, after he had shattered the sail-racing world with *Avenger*, Uffa deplored the abandonment of the heavy plate . . . but we must not stray too far from the main thread.

From those days in the 1920s we have now reached a time when many classes of these high power-to-weight ratio racing dinghies turn out in their thousands every weekend. Because they carry a large amount of sail they can readily be thrown on their beam-ends or capsized. But that's all part of the fun. Thrills and spills. And the boats have built-in buoyancy, while their crews have tied-on buoyancy, and are in any case skilled at righting their boats, bailing them out and getting them sailing again. Nowadays it is part of every sailing school's curriculum to teach capsize and righting drill – so much so that people who come new to sailing are led to believe that capsizing is a natural and inevitable part of the sport. And that is very regrettable, because it is just not true.

A man and a woman set out for an afternoon's sail from Poole in a sailing dinghy. Lured on by the sunshine, they sailed out of the harbour, past the Old Harry rock, speeded

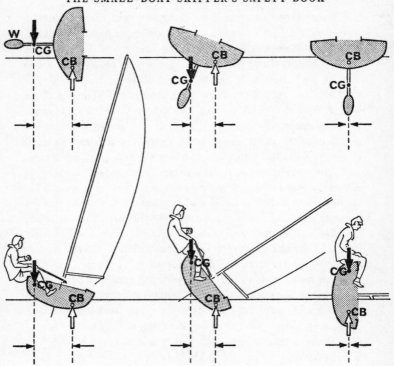

The difference between a ballast-keel boat and a 'human-ballast' dinghy. The keel-boat's ballast puts her centre of gravity well down, and the maximum righting leverage is when she is on her beam ends. As she comes more upright both the CG and the CB move inward, and the righting moment is nil when she is upright and both centres are in the same vertical line.

In the lower strip, CG and CB are farthest apart (and the righting leverage is greatest) when the boat is only slightly heeled – enough to move CB away from centre-line. As angle of heel increases, righting leverage decreases. It reaches a minimum when she is on her beam-ends.

southward into a freshening wind by the ebb tide. Somewhere towards Swanage in steepening seas they capsized, and like the competent crew they were they soon righted the boat and had her sailing again. But now they were getting into the overfalls of the shoal off Peveril Point and they capsized again. They were a little slower to right her this time, and in a few moments they were over again. The story as pieced together by the Coastguard does not say how many times they capsized, but perhaps twice more as they became colder, more tired, and less agile. Each time they remained longer in the water and were carried farther south towards Durleston Head. When they were finally spotted by the Coastguard station there they had given up trying to right the boat – they had little strength left, and all they could do was to hang on and hope.

That couple had the wrong boat for the sort of excursion they wanted to make. It is one thing to capsize while racing round the buoys, not too far from the club house, and with the safety boat in attendance, but it is not something to be taken lightly when you are at sea, and on your own. It is true that some people can get away with it, just as some people climb Mont Blanc, but it is foolish to suppose that what one or two exceptionally hardy and well-trained people can do is a model for imitation by the rest of us ordinary folk.

This is what I call the 'other kind of dinghy', though some people would look at it the other way round. Let us say that there are some open sailing boats which look after their crews, whereas there are others which demand to be looked after. This second category is the racing dinghy, which is kept up by the agility of the people on board, which may yet go over, and then wait for those same people to put her back on her feet again. One cannot even be complacent about the racing dinghy when she *is* with the rest of the bunch, in an organised event with the safety boat in attendance. Every year the lifeboats are called out to multiple capsizes when so many boats go over in a few seconds that the club safety boat cannot cope. This is what it looks like in the RNLI's report:

Llandudno. At 1250 the local sailing club requested assistance for the club's guard boats in a race in which several sailing dinghies had capsized in squally weather off Little Orme's Head. The Inshore Rescue Boat was launched at 1300 in a strong south-westerly offshore wind with a rough sea. . . . she was followed five minutes later by the lifeboat *Lily Wainwright*. The lifeboat came up with the first dinghy at 1315, took off her crew of two and took the dinghy in tow. She then located three other dinghies, righted them and took them in tow. The IRB found two further dinghies which had beached in Whitechapel Bay and towed them to Llandudno Bay. The tug *Elizabeth Howard* marked one further dinghy about 6 to 7 miles offshore as it was a danger to shipping. When all crews had been reported safe, the IRB returned to her station at 1600 and the lifeboat at 1835.

Quite a good bag for one afternoon's work, and please don't think that I have picked on a rarity – multiple capsizes and multiple rescues abound during every sailing season. It is something worth remembering when one reads that the RNLI has rescued large numbers of 'yachtsmen' during the year, for you may think (as I do) that on some of these occasions the club's officers should not have allowed racing to be held. Or one may take the view that the wrong type of boat has been adopted by a club for those particular waters.

Unfortunately there is no simple way of defining the characteristics of the boat that will look after you as opposed to the boat that you must look after. But in any case before I stick my neck out on that tricky distinction there are one or two points that should be made on the subject of the 'capsizable' type of boat. The first is to draw attention to the importance of keeping all the loose gear attached to the boat so that it cannot come free and drift away. One still hears of such things as the loss of a rudder after a capsize, in spite of the fact that it could have been secured with a simple lanyard, or with one of the patent nylon spring gadgets that are sold especially for the purpose. The bailer, centreboard, paddle (oars are better) and so forth must all obviously be attached to the boat.

Another point that is often overlooked is that it is not uncommon for one of the crew to become so entangled with the rigging that he becomes powerless to right the boat or to clamber back aboard. It sounds unlikely if you have not experienced it, but it does happen.

The type of boat which is expected to capsize will almost certainly be fitted with buoyancy, and for some owners there is the temptation to fit extra buoyancy just to be on the safe side. But too much buoyancy can be a great hindrance, for it lifts the boat higher out of the water and makes her more difficult to right. Furthermore, the extra windage increases the rate of drift, which is a very undesirable thing. I think that nowadays nearly everybody has had dinned into them the message that if the boat cannot be righted the proper thing to do is to stay with her. Obviously if you are a good swimmer and safety really is only a few yards away you would be right to swim for it. But it can be done only if you are absolutely certain of success, and as a general rule it *is* far better to stay with the boat. It not only offers support, but also makes an easily visible target for the rescue service when it sets out. A human head in the sea is a very difficult thing to spot.

THE SEAWORTHY FAMILY DINGHY

Safety apart, there are many people who want to go for a day's sail without the risk of a capsize. They want to be sure that their camera and picnic gear will not be soaked with water, that their spare clothes will remain dry and that their children will not be frightened. They may think that a family outing in comfort and peace of mind is more to be desired than a few exhilarating minutes of high-speed planing. Fortunately that type of sailing is still possible, there are plenty of boats which will look after you if you use only a reasonable amount of common sense. I have watched a friend of mine sailing year after year in his clinker-built *Yachting World* Dayboat, taking her to sea in squally weather and sailing serenely on while racing dinghies were capsizing around him in their dozens. To the best of my knowledge he has never capsized his boat, though he has sailed her in all weathers.

That record is a tribute to his common sense and good seamanship, but it is also a tribute to the boat. He could easily have done the same in other boats of the 'right' type, but it would have been much harder in boats of the 'wrong' type. And *right* and *wrong* in this context relate only to the intended use of the boat – either kind is equally right if used for the right purpose, in the right waters and under the right conditions. The difficulty is to find some way of sorting t'other from which . . .

The first thing one can do is to try to get a feeling for the underlying factors which contribute to stability. It is evident that a fairly heavy boat, with plenty of beam and relatively little sail area will be less easy to capsize than a lighter, narrower craft which is carrying more sail area. It is also obvious, as has already been said a few paragraphs back, that a deep and heavy keel has a good restoring effect just at the moment when it is most needed – when the boat is near the point when her mast will go in the water.

But one cannot simply give a ratio of beam to length, for example, and say that a dinghy with such and such a ratio is

'safe' while another proportion is not, because the hull of a
boat is a complex shape and a figure taken at one point is not
much indication of the whole form. One might, for example,
say that if a 10-foot stem dinghy has a beam of less than 4½ feet
amidships one may logically begin to wonder if she will be of
the right sort to look after you. That would be a starting point,
but nothing more. And one would have to take a different
figure as the starting point for a boat of different length, though
the *proportion* would be very much the same for general-
purpose dinghies in the range from 8 to about 16 feet in
length.

And that is not the whole story, for the kind of boat that
needs to be looked after will have a very similar ratio of mid-
ships beam to length *at the deck or gunwale level*. Where she is
likely to differ is in having less beam at the waterline, but
waterline beam is a figure that is not usually given in the
brochures, nor is it easily checked.

In practice one has to solve the problem by gathering clues
of all kinds. One obvious thing to do is to ask some people
who ought to know, and I say 'some' because there is always
the risk that you will be talking to someone who either has some
bee in his bonnet, or who lacks real knowledge. One can ask
a sailing school, or get in touch with the Dinghy Cruising
Association whose members do know from experience which
types of boat look after their occupants. One can use one's own
eyes. Boats which are fitted with toe-straps, sliding seats,
trapezes, and other gadgets which allow the crew to use their
body weight with maximum leverage to keep the boat upright,
automatically reveal their true nature. Boats that look as if you
are expected to sit *in* them rather than to perch *on* the edge are
less likely to lead you into trouble. Broadly speaking boats
which are much used for racing are in fact racing boats. Boats
which are little used for racing are more sedate.

Magazine reports are a useful guide, especially if you are sufficiently perceptive to detect any special enthusiasm in the writer that may colour his report. And there's no law that prevents you from writing to a magazine for advice, though as one who is at the receiving end of many questions I can say quite bluntly that the inquirer *must* give a clear indication of the sort of use he envisages for the boat.

There is one type of evidence that is often suspect, and that is the kind which says 'Bill Bloggs sailed one across the Channel, so she must be a good dinghy . . .' That is bad logic, and it is even worse when some manufacturer organises a stunt voyage to draw attention to his product. It is not unknown for a boatbuilder to organise some such trip for a dozen or so little boats, with launches in attendance and so forth. The trip may have to be postponed for bad weather, but you won't hear of that, for the announcement will only be made when at last a successful trip is made. This kind of thing is in fact quite irresponsible, because the innocent newcomer to boats may see the newspaper report that makes it all sound so easy, and be tempted to try and follow suit. Sailing alone, with no escort, and minimum experience, he is a candidate for Davy Jones's locker.

In contrast to the stunt passage is the genuine performer. There is the chap like Frank Dye, for example, who some years ago showed that long sea trips could be made in an open dinghy, and the fact that he chose a *Wayfarer* for the job was clear evidence for the seaworthiness of that particular design – not because she carried him so far, but because he (as a man of experience) chose her for that job. Nor did his exploits, among which was the sailing of that 16-foot open boat from Scotland to Norway via the Faroes in really severe conditions, make any justification for others to conclude that by buying a similar boat they could do the same. One can buy a pair of climbing-boots but whether one can climb the Matterhorn is another matter.

In this attempt to define the indefinable, and to warn people against trying to use a racing dinghy for solitary seagoing, I am very much aware that there is a middle ground occupied by certain designs which are widely raced but are also tolerably good seaboats. The *Mirror* and the *Gull* come into that category, for example, while there are also boats such as the *Salcombe Yawl* which are fine for the sea, and are also raced though they are not 'racing boats'. And let us not put all the blame on the boat. Sail area can be reduced, or, if it cannot, then that boat is automatically debarred as far as I am concerned. And there is the decision whether to go out at all, even with reduced sail.

OPEN LAUNCHES AND RUNABOUTS

Although this chapter has been concerned about open sailing dinghies, and their performance on the sea (or on lakes where the wind has a long enough fetch to make the water rough) it might be worth saying a few words about open launches and runabouts. Small open power craft are not likely to be capsized, except in extreme conditions, because they do not suffer the heeling force of sails. But in certain sea conditions they can take water over the side – and especially over the bow and transom. It is the short confused sea that causes most trouble, and that is found where a tide runs over shallows, or where big rollers come into shoal water. Both these conditions are likely to be met at harbour mouths and river estuaries, which are much more likely to endanger small craft than the open sea a few miles offshore.

In artificial harbours there is another dangerous type of wave pattern, caused by reflections of waves from solid stone walls. As with other harbour-mouth disturbances the insidious danger arises when a boat which has been at sea returns in search of shelter. She may come back because the open-sea conditions were becoming too rough for comfort – only to find conditions even worse as she makes the final approach and entrance to her haven of refuge.

Probably the greatest danger to small power craft, and especially to fast runabouts and ski-boats is mis-handling by the helmsman. That is really a matter of seamanship, and a subject for a separate book. But it can be said in general terms that, as with sailing dinghies, a small fast boat should not be used in inappropriate conditions. And if conditions are rough then care must be taken with the speed, the trim and the direction of the boat. Too much speed, or weight too much aft can result in a 'flip' or somersault. On the other hand, a sudden closing of the throttle (perhaps because of the approach of an especially menacing wave) may drop the bow so that it dips and shovels water back into the cockpit. The importance of direction is that seas may sometimes be made more comfortable if taken at an angle, so lessening their steepness.

The driver of a fast runabout or ski-boat has more to consider than his own safety. There are others, especially bathers and passengers, to whom he may cause serious injury if he is careless. Without doubt the most frightening thing about a small high-speed craft in the vicinity of a bathing beach is the sharp-edged spinning propeller, which in most such boats is completely exposed. There is a steady growth in the appeal of jet-propelled boats, whose greatest merit, in my view, is their real contribution to safety. As the waters become more and more crowded I hope that we may see more and more jet boats coming into service, for that one reason. Although 'jet' has a connotation of speed deriving from its aeronautical applications, a jet-propelled boat is no faster than a screw-boat of the same power. In fact it tends to be fractionally slower. But it has great advantages in shallow water which, added to its safety, make it ideal for sport and ski-ing use.

A final point that is worth making concerns care where propellers are concerned. Every summer I see small craft with children perched on their bows, dangling their feet in the water, or even being towed alongside. A slip, or a slight error of judgement could result in terrible injuries from the propeller, yet there are always a few people whose imagination has not yet reached that far.

In the same way, there are always a few people who have not yet cottoned on to the fact that, unlike a car, a boat steers by swinging her back end. So if somebody falls into the water on the port side of the boat, the helmsman must instantly turn her to port, thus swinging the stern away to starboard – away from the victim.

Another danger that is met in very fast runabouts is their ability to throw the driver out of the boat and into the water. It happens when the going is rough, and then one may be faced with a driverless craft careering off on its own at about 30 m.p.h. – a terrifying experience, not least for the driver now in the water, if the boat happens to circle back. But that situation can easily be avoided by a safety cut-out to the ignition, linked to a line which is attached to the driver's clothing or life-jacket. Ready-made devices can be bought from chandlers' shops, or a marine engineer will rig one up to order. It is neither complex nor costly.

One last word about small, outboard-powered boats. In the experience of the RNLI their capsize fatality rate is unusually high. So all that has been said about fitting buoyancy to the boat and wearing it yourself has special significance. And one must be specially careful to avoid any chance of capsize.

10. Trouble With Tenders

Most experienced yachtsmen will tell you that more people are drowned while trying to get to or from their boats in the dinghy than in any other circumstances. I don't think that there are any actual figures to support such a claim, but you don't have to be around long before you realise that too many people are drowned each year as a result of accidents in yachts' tenders, and the reason is not hard to find. *They are too small.*

An open rowing boat, even a small open rowing boat when that word is used in its ordinary sense, can carry three or four people in quite a chop and still remain seaworthy. But the yacht's tender is even smaller than that (to augment imprecision with further imprecision). You see them every season – a tiny boat which may be packed to overflowing with people, and perhaps with their gear. She has very little freeboard, and because she is carrying such a large weight in proportion to her immersed volume she is dead in her movements and does not lift readily to the sea. Thus it won't take much of a wave to slop some water over her bow – even more likely it will come in over the stern and make somebody's bottom wet, which is good for a giggle unless . . . Unless he or she fidgets and upsets the whole caboodle. There just isn't any room for fidgeting in a tiny boat so overladen – there probably is not even room for one of the crew to get a bailer down between the tangle of legs and start scooping some of the water out. In fact the whole thing is plain bloody dangerous.

Yet every year it happens all over again, and some family suffers a tragedy. The root of the problem lies in the fact that the cruising boat has to take her tender away with her and she wants the smallest possible boat, whether she is going to tow it, or stow it on deck. And the skipper wants the smallest possible boat because every so often he and his crew are going to have to drag her up or down a beach.

Various solutions have been found to this problem, among them the folding canvas boat and the inflatable. A well-made inflatable (in contrast to the much cheaper 'beach toy' type of thing) offers stability, ample reserve buoyancy, the ability to fold up into a small space for stowage and light weight for lifting ashore or on board. On the other hand she is a pig to row, and offers little in the way of comfort to those who occupy her. Nevertheless, when one hears of a tragedy involving a yacht's tender it is most unlikely to be an inflatable. No, the boats that cause the trouble are 7- and 8-foot solid dinghies, often prams, built in marine plywood or glass-reinforced resin. And since it is evident that people still use these tiny boats in large numbers one must simply suggest that all possible precautions be taken.

And perhaps the first need is to be sure that such boats have sufficient built-in buoyancy not only to keep themselves afloat but also to provide 20 to 30 pounds for each occupant – something in the order of $\frac{1}{2}$ cubic foot for each person. A flooded wooden boat will do more than support herself. If built in agba ply, for example, she will offer about 9 lb *excess* buoyancy for every 10 lb of her own weight, but if built in the more durable makore she would give between 5 lb and 6 lb surplus buoyancy for each 10 lb of her own weight. A plywood dinghy weighing 100 lb may, in broad terms, support not only herself when filled with water but something between 50 and 90 lb weight of material.

A resin-glass dinghy, on the other hand, will not even be able to support her own weight unless she has special buoyancy. The resin-glass laminations in a dinghy would have a density of about 95 lb per cubic foot which is about half as much again as water at 60 lb/cu.ft. That is why virtually all resin-glass dinghies are built with integral buoyancy compartments, for it is in fact laid down by the Ship and Boatbuilders National Federation that a dinghy should *at least* be able to support her own weight when filled with water. If one has a dinghy with hollow buoyancy spaces it is a good idea to fill them with polyurethane foam, or even with plastic bottles, or pingpong balls, for one can never be quite sure that one of these spaces does not have a tiny leak.

If extra buoyancy in the form of inflated bags, empty chemical bottles, copper tanks or the like is to be fitted into a dinghy, it is important that it be fixed *very firmly*. It is remarkable with what force a buoyant container will burst its way out of a partially submerged boat.

And having provided oneself with a dinghy which will keep her occupants afloat even after she has tipped them in, it would be logical to ensure that she has some kind of handholds. Tired, cold hands cannot get much of a grip on the smooth bottom of a plastic dinghy, however well she herself may be floating.

Having seen to the buoyancy it would be as well, if one

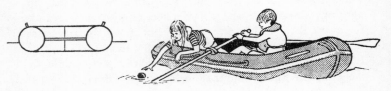

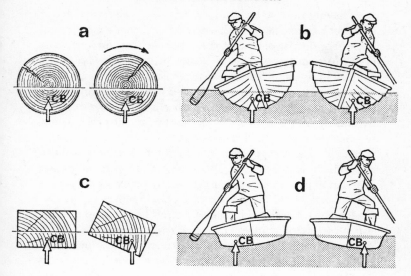

The stability of a dinghy is influenced by her cross-sectional shape and the way the centre of buoyancy moves when she heels. A round log, **a**, can heel *ad infinitum* without any effect on the CB. A round-bottomed boat, **b**, is somewhat similar but the flare in the upper parts of the hull provides buoyancy as it dips, and so the CB moves under the man.

A rectangular log, **c**, returns from a heeled position because the CB moves to one side (the CB is the centre of the immersed area). A boat with a more nearly rectangular section moves her CB a long way for a small angle of heel, as may be seen by comparing immersed areas in **b** and **d**.

The typical inflatable dinghy seen opposite is very nearly rectangular in section and so tends to be stable. The round buoyancy tubes have no effect on the movement of the CB which is dependent only on the outer form of the hull, but they make it almost impossible to put one's weight at the extreme beam of the boat. In short they tend to keep people in the middle.

were buying from scratch to look for one which has plenty of beam and a cross-sectional shape that is virtually a rectangle. It is the wide, flat bottom of the inflatable boats (at least most of them) that makes them so stable. Although it is a rather childish over-simplification, one may liken a boat to an ornament standing on the mantelpiece – if it stands on a broad flat base it is not likely to topple over when a heavy lorry rumbles by outside. But if it stands on a narrow base and widens out towards the top . . . well it's obvious.

Stability can be appraised in a dinghy by seeing how far to one side it is possible to stand, and that is an important criterion in practice because many dinghy accidents are caused when a member of the party stands up and moves to one side to step aboard a bigger boat or a jetty. The situation is made worse by the thoughtless or inexperienced person who *pushes* downward with a foot near the edge of the dinghy instead of pulling himself up. But even when such a person is doing his best to make a mess of things, those still in the dinghy can help by taking an active part in the balancing and steadying of the boat and not just sitting there like dummies until they are tipped in. Designers of the bigger boats can help too, and so can owners, by providing steps of some kind so that one can step aboard easily and securely from a dinghy. I believe that most of these 'transfer' accidents could be eliminated if the step from dinghy to boat were not such a taxing one, especially for women who are generally shorter in the leg and less muscular in their arms than men. Incidentally, I notice that a woman is often unwilling to be parted from her handbag, even for the moment of transfer. But it is better that the step be made empty-handed: bags and other bits and bobs can be passed up afterwards.

Within a given length, and as we have said most yachts' tenders *are* very small, the pram shape has the advantage, for it carries the beam well forward. A stem dinghy, with pointed bow, offers very little resistance to heeling if a man steps forward. The beamier mid- and after-sections tend to lift up out of the water so that they have little stabilising effect, and the narrow bow dips in and rolls over. Weight, too, is a great contributor to stability, since it is the weight of the boat herself that has to counterbalance the weight of a man standing to one side. In that condition the two weights are balancing about the centre of buoyancy of the boat. But people want light dinghies, just as they want small ones . . .

What they ought not to put up with is too little freeboard, which is a not infrequent fault among prams. We had a plywood pram at one time of a very popular type, about 8 feet long. She would take three people out the couple of hundred yards to our mooring, but a slight lop or the wash of a passing boat, and water would start slopping over the quarters or amidships. By the rather crude procedure of gluing and screwing a 3-inch strip of plywood all round the top I made her into twice the boat, and we never had any trouble thereafter. Yet there are hundreds of these boats in use – I see them everywhere, and I wonder how their owners manage.

Such boats are easily over-driven under the power of an outboard. If the dinghy is heavily laden and the motor is opened up, water may surge in over the bow transom, and the thing may bury her nose and plunge like a submarine. I saw a classical example of it one sunny evening, but it happened among the moorings with plenty of boats to come to the rescue, so mum, dad, granny and two infants were quickly fished out of the water. Getting the boat and her heavy motor up from the bottom took longer, though. A year later, and after the above words had been written, I saw the whole thing repeated on the same stretch of water by a different couple, also coming ashore on Sunday evening in a very small pram. Under the power of the outboard she was pushing up a curling bow-wave, and only a small ripple was needed to raise it the extra inch to start flowing over the bow-transom. Coming ashore in a sailing dinghy we could see what was likely to happen, and that if the water once started running over the bow the process would accelerate as she tripped over her own bow.

'Just like that dinghy last year,' we said to each other, but we could not make the couple hear because of the noise of their motor. And the husband could not see what was happening under his bow because his wife was sitting in the line of sight; and she was facing aft. There were plenty of people around, so when they did go down the result was an annoyance rather than a catastrophe. But that couple must have wondered what might have followed a similar event on a dark, cold night . . .

A jolly little clinker pram about 6 feet long that we used to own could easily be over-driven under oars, even when lightly laden, as I found on one winter's day when I heard a cry for help. The water was choppy, and rowing as fast as I could I quickly had my own boat half-full of water. There were nearly two people crying for help, that day!

A small dinghy is best with something of no more than $1\frac{1}{2}$ or 2 h.p., though engine power may permissibly grow rapidly as the boat is longer than 10 feet. But for a tender the smallest motors, weighing only about 20 lb, are best.

Every dinghy should carry a bailer of course, attached to the boat by a lanyard, so that it cannot be lost overboard. It is important not to allow water to accumulate in the bottom of the boat because it becomes a *mobile mass* which will move instantly downhill. So, if you shift your weight slightly to one side, perhaps by missing your footing, the weight of water will also move down to that side and make matters worse. It is the opposite of the corrective action you would wish to have.

But one always comes back to the fact that overloading is the main source of trouble, often associated with the obvious fact that people tend to be less careful when they come out of a bar after an evening's jollification. And darkness makes it all so much worse. It is easier for someone to miss his footing, easier for the oarsman to get the boat across somebody else's mooring chain (which may lead to instant capsize if a strong stream is running), and harder to find survivors if they should go into the water. It follows that the wise skipper will fix a maximum number that the dinghy may carry, even if somebody does have to wait ashore in the rain. And the only exception he will make is to *reduce* the number when visibility is bad, the wind is strong, the water choppy, or when any circumstance gives the least cause for doubt.

One afternoon I saw a chap sit in his dinghy for an hour, made fast to a mooring half way between his boat and the shore – a mere hundred yards either way. He had found that he simply could not pull the boat against the combined force of wind and tide, so there he had to stay until somebody chanced by in a motor launch. Had he thought about it, he could have tested the water, so to speak, by bending an extra length of rope to his painter and trying his luck before finally casting off.

Incidentally, it is noteworthy that this chap was alone in his boat. Had he had the extra weight and windage of a couple of passengers his situation would have been far worse. And that gives me a chance to air one of the bats in my own belfry: if there is more than one person in a dinghy, then more than one should be able to row. People represent horsepower, and there's no point in having unused power that is so much deadweight. Even an 8-foot pram will usually allow two rowing positions, though few people seem to bother to carry the second pair of oars and rowlocks. If the pram cannot be trimmed for two people to pull, then one person must sit in the sternsheets and push-row. It is not the easiest way, but the work load is shared, and the progress will show a marked difference. If there are three people, then one can go aft and the other two can pull from the bow and centre thwarts. Many people who go to the expense of buying an outboard, and the trouble of looking after it, could be happier and healthier if they arranged to make use of the human horsepower that is available.

There are also good safety reasons for having two pairs of oars and rowlocks in a boat, especially if children are allowed to row about on their own. Everybody loses an oar over the side sooner or later; then follows the attempt to grab it which may result in a capsize. Alternatively it may stay out of reach, and then the boat will drift at the mercy of wind and current, unless she is equipped for anchoring or the person on board is skilled in wangling or sculling with a single oar over the transom. (It is an art which is learned easily enough once you know that the oar should be held with the wrist beneath it.)

But it is not only a matter of dropping an oar overboard. I could cite the example of the three men in a motor boat who anchored off Corriegravie, near Campbeltown when their motor broke down. They rowed ashore in the dinghy so that one of the party could go to seek help. The other two set off back to the boat with the idea of having another go at the engine, but half way out one of their oars broke, and as there was a strong easterly blowing they began to 'sail' out to sea at a fine rate of knots. Fortunately they were seen, and another lifeboat call was chalked up on the score-board.

There are times when it is wise to take a compass with you in your tender. One can lose one's way on a dark night, even in familiar waters, and in fog or mist it is even easier. An anchor, on the other hand should always be carried, with a cable somewhat longer than the boat's painter. A routine report by the RNLI station at Harwich underlines the point:

At 1628 . . . news was received that a dinghy with a crew of
two had set out from the beach to join the yacht *Solent
Sprite*, but high winds had swept the dinghy to the other
side of the harbour . . .

And another one, from RNLI at Eastney in Hampshire:

At about 1600 it was learned that a rowing dinghy with three
people on board had been swept out to sea from Langstone
Harbour . . . it was half an hour after high water and the
current was very strong . . .

And from Selsey in Sussex:

. . . the Coastguard reported that a rowing dinghy with two
men on board was in difficulties about 1 mile south-west of
Selsey Bill. At 1310 the Inshore Rescue Boat was launched
. . . The IRB came up with the dinghy, which had lost an
oar, as it was being swept out to sea on the receding tide.

One could go on quoting little stories like these. They fill
pages of the lifeboatmen's reports every year, and so often the
provision of a second pair of oars or an anchor would have
made all the difference.

I suppose that we are all guilty at some time or other of
neglecting some little details, and I would not wish to give the
impression that I consider myself beyond reproach and therefore entitled to lecture everybody else. Even though one may
be perfectly prepared in one respect there is likely to be some
deficiency in another quarter. And there is also that fatal and
insidious thought, 'it will be alright this time – I'll do something
about it next time . . .'

I can quote my own neglect as an example of that type of
delusion. Our present mooring is a good way from the hard
where we launch the dinghy, so far that I succumbed to the

temptation to buy an outboard motor to help us when the tide is foul – for even under power it is a fifteen-minute run at the least. At the beginning of the season I was perfectly aware that I had not brought the dinghy anchor out of store, yet subconsciously I *felt* that it was still only the beginning of the season, and that the game hadn't really started yet . . . Sheer folly, of course, as we found when a gale blew down the creek with the ebb tide as we were trying to go home. It was raining of course, and then the outboard began to play up: it would run for a few minutes and then stop. Each time we got it started again we had drifted back to square one. Although I had not brought the anchor, we did have our usual two pairs of oars on board, but even with both of us rowing we could make no headway against the strong tide and the wind. All we could do was to hold our own. In the end we gave up, fell back to the boat and brewed up, while I tried (and failed) to trace the fault in the motor. Finally we had to wait until the ebb had finished and when the flood was running well we were able to row up against the wind. We got home about five hours later than we had planned, and about five hours later than we should have done if we had had an anchor to hold the ground we could gain from short bursts of the motor, or short hard bursts on the oars. (In the good light and leisure of the garage at home I found the little piece of dirt in the fuel system that had been causing the trouble.)

A last, and some may think a rather fanciful, point about yachts' tenders concerns the unsuspected leak at night. Everybody knows that a clinker dinghy which has been left to dry out in the sun is likely to open up and leak furiously when she is first put into the water. (Which is why it is best to store a clinker dinghy right way up so that she will hold rainwater and stay damp.)

Now what happens when you come down on Friday night and set off in the dark, having loaded (even *over*loaded) the boat with people and stores, and a couple of hundred yards from shore you notice a cold clammy feeling around your ankles . . .?

The first time it happened to me was a long time ago, when I was a boy and with a friend I was given the job of taking out stores. It happened again some thirty years later, when I should have known better, and all because I had stowed a clinker dinghy upside down on the quay in a hot summer.

A similar thing happened again a few years later with a plywood boat which had been left on the quay. What we did not notice when we arrived in the dark was that somebody had knocked a hole in her bottom. It may have been mischief, or just bad judgement in backing a car. Now this boat was divided into two separate compartments by a watertight bulkhead amidships, and it was our practice to load all stores into the forward half, and ourselves into the after half. In that pitch dark it was quite a time before we discovered that the front half was 9 inches deep in water. No danger of course because that boat had so much buoyancy built into her, but we lost some cameras, a radio set, and most of our food.

Now I take care to make an inspection before launching a dinghy into the water in the dark – and another after she's in. Next time it will be some other unexpected thing that will catch me out, but each time one learns another lesson. At least one ought to. The lesson I have learned is to make sure that the tender has a good strong towing eye, fitted low down, and a painter strong enough for the boat to be towed when laden. An extra length of rope for use with the anchor may come in handy in other ways, of course. I insist on having at least one spare oar and rowlock, and normally carry two. Each rowlock is attached to the boat by a lanyard. Built-in buoyancy, securely fitted, is also on my own list and should be on every-body's, I think. When I am using an outboard, then a can of fuel and a minimum tool kit always go with it wherever it goes. Such things are obvious, but each skipper must consider the matter in the light of his own circumstances, and there are occasions when even a tender should carry more elaborate gear (a torch by night for example, or a compass). In Chapter 14 I list many items which may be needed on any boat, be she large or small, according to circumstances.

11. Little Boats Should Be Seen . . .

For many people the most frightening thing about going to sea is the possibility of being run down by a large ship. It is easy for the imagination to throw up gruesome pictures, especially when one has seen the bows-on view of one or two ships at rather close quarters. There is something menacing about the bulk of a ship – so much so that some people find it hard to believe that an approaching vessel is not motivated by some malicious intent.

All such panicky feelings must be suppressed when it comes to a real situation, for careful observation and detached thought will be absolutely necessary if the right decision is to be made. A ship may seem to be absolutely head-on to a nervous member of your crew, until you are able to point out that her masts are not in line, or that it is possible to see down one side of her hull but not the other. And by night the arrangement of a ship's lights gives a very good indication of her attitude in relation to your own craft, so the wise owner will make a careful study of light patterns before undertaking any night passages. As with so many other aspects of safety we are entering into the realms of general seamanship, which is a proper subject for a separate book.

Although ships look so menacing on some occasions, and although one must treat them as a serious threat, running down

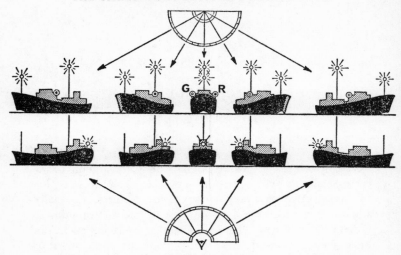

Coming or going, a ship's attitude is indicated by her masts, her hull shape, and her lights. The bow-wave and wash are more subtle, yet useful, indications. The after mast and light are always higher than the forward ones. At night, as she steams by, her side-light (red or green) will be seen from dead ahead through an angle of $112\frac{1}{2}°$: in other words to $22\frac{1}{2}°$ aft of the beam. The two masthead lights show through the same angle. As these three lights are cut off, the single white stern light will become visible – provided that all is correctly adjusted.

of private craft does not seem to be a very common occurrence. Big ships seem to collide more frequently with each other than with their tiny sisters, perhaps because we who are in the little craft are sufficiently frightened to take special care. It is true that each year a few yachts 'disappear' while on passage, and that for want of a better explanation some of these losses are attributed to running down. But the number is small, and it can be kept so if skippers of small craft take suitable precautions.

LITTLE BOATS SHOULD BE SEEN ...

KEEPING A LOOK-OUT

The first and most important of these is to keep a good look-out. It is unwise to assume that the crew of a big ship, assisted by radar and supposedly watching from a comfortable and sheltered position high above the water, will spot your little craft and keep clear. Many do, of course, but there are some whose standards of seamanship are lower than yours and mine, and who leave the ship on automatic pilot while they do Heaven-knows-what below decks: these are the people who cause worry to the skippers of small boats – and to the masters of big ships ...

Obviously, the party who is likely to suffer most in a collision is the one who must keep alert. Some experienced small-boat seamen even go so far as to say that it is better not to try to draw attention to oneself with bright lights and a radar reflector. A pedestrian, the argument runs, does not light himself up and then wander about the road hoping that drivers will dodge him–he watches for the lights of the cars and keeps well out of their way until the road is clear.

In effect, most small-boat skippers do just that, but there seems no gain in *not* carrying the prescribed lights and the best possible radar reflector. In fact, I am firmly of the opinion that it is important and valuable to do so, and I shall have some more to say on that matter. For the moment a few words more on the subject of keeping a sharp look-out.

On a long passage, especially when one is huddled against cold or rain in an open cockpit and eyes are tired from sun and spray, it is quite natural to settle down into a comatose mood, watching only the compass and the set of the sails, or to succumb to the drone of the engine. In such conditions the threat from astern may be forgotten – yet with ships moving at four or five times the speed of one's own boat the overtaking situation is a very likely source of danger. With sufficient crew the problem is eased, because one member can be deputed to keep watch astern, leaving the helmsman to look ahead, as is natural for him. But for the single-hander, or the usual husband-and-wife team, a conscious effort and a personal drill are required to ensure that all quarters of the horizon are scanned every few minutes.

Just how often the horizon must be scanned depends on the visibility and the location. On a clear night, when ships' lights may be seen several miles away it is evidently a much less rigorous business than on a misty afternoon, or in a heavy rainstorm. Furthermore, ships tend to keep to fairly well-defined lanes, and in busy waters such as the English Channel one may go for long periods without seeing any shipping, and then for a period of an hour or so there will be a steady procession of them all steaming up or down Channel to their next turning mark. When clear of these lanes one can relax somewhat, but unless you are on ocean passage out in the Atlantic, there is always the odd ship on some out-of-the ordinary passage and one must still maintain a good watch.

When visibility falls to less than half a mile, say, a small boat fitted with a good radar reflector should be able to cross the shipping lanes without ever seeing a large vessel. With their radar, ships' officers should see us and steer clear so that they never come within visual range . . . which is why people sometimes come in after a passage in thick weather and report that there 'seemed to be no ships about'. Perhaps it is true that what the eye doesn't see the heart does not grieve, but on the whole I make my passages in good visibility for choice, and in bad visibility only by chance.

LIGHTS

This is not the place to give details of the lights that each kind of vessel must show after dark: one assumes that such things are already known to the boat owner, for they are readily available in a variety of publications ranging from *Reed's Almanac* to my own *Small Boat Cruising*. The practical problem with most yachts is that lights must be mounted rather low, where they can easily be obscured by high seas, and that the electrical supply is often severely limited. The battery capacity is usually the critical factor for a sailing boat, and that tempts boatbuilders and owners to fit rather low-powered bulbs. Now although the Collision Regulations make special provision for small craft and allow their lights to be visible over shorter distances than those of big ships, it is evident that many private craft have lights too feeble even to reach out to that reduced distance (i.e. 1 mile for the red and green and 3 miles for the white forward light on power craft; 2 miles for the white stern light). Taking into account the high speed and scandalously poor controllability of some modern ships, one can only say that we all need the brightest lights we can possibly fit.

In saying that, one has to appreciate that coloured glasses absorb between 85 and 90 per cent of the light that comes from the bulb, so that it is far harder to get a satisfactory performance with the port and starboard lamps than with the white lights which show forward and aft.

In effect this is saying that the light through a white glass is 8 times brighter than it is through a red or green one, but that does not mean that it will be detectable by the human eye at 8 times the distance. The proportion is nearer the square root of 8 in practice. And without going too deeply into the physics of the matter that leads us to the point that beyond a visibility of a mile or two very large increases in bulb wattage will be needed to obtain even small increments in range of visibility. For example, to increase the visibility from 3 miles to 4 would call for a lamp twice as bright.

In practice, those of us who sail around in small craft cannot expect to have lamps which will be visible at such distances. A 24-watt, 12-volt bulb showing through clear glass would have a visibility of about 3 miles in good conditions, and only a slight deterioration in the clarity of the atmosphere would reduce that range to 2 miles or less.

A bulb of the same wattage behind good quality coloured glass or Perspex would be visible at a bit more than 1 mile in good conditions (though probably not at $1\frac{1}{2}$ miles) and it would be correspondingly less in haze, mist or rain. There is one gain that can be made with the coloured lights. Since we have to show red to port and green to starboard it is possible to use a single lamp with a bi-colour glass, and that lamp can be of double the wattage that one could afford for each of two single lamps. (In effect one is making use of light that would otherwise be lost inside the lamp-housing, for the lamps made for boats are not yet provided with properly-designed and optically efficient reflectors.)

In theory, which is not always the same as in practice, a white stern light of 12w gives a clear-night visibility of nearly 2 miles, while a bi-colour lamp with a 36w bulb should give about $1\frac{3}{4}$ miles. A 48w lamp in the bi-colour would bring its visibility nearer to 2 miles, or approximately the same as the white stern light.

Assuming that we are still talking of a 12-volt system, and remembering that $amps \times volts = watts$, we can say that the current flow will be 4 or 5 amps, depending on whether the total wattage of the navigation lights amounts to 50w or 60w. Ignoring any other demands on the battery, such as compass light, the implication is that for a summer night of eight hours' darkness one must have a battery with a minimum capacity of 40 amp-hours, and most people would double that to feel comfortable. It is important not to forget that the battery may be needed for engine-starting as well.

It is conceivable that other forms of lamp could be used where electricity is not abundant. The very bright luminous mantle of the Tilley paraffin pressure lamp, or the more compact version of the same thing which runs from a small bottle of liquefied gas might be adapted for the purpose. But there are many practical problems, and I would think it unlikely that such lamps will ever go into commercial production, though a clever handyman might make his own.

Although a bi-colour lamp makes the best use of a limited amount of radiant energy, it does have two disadvantages. The fact that the red and green are so close together means that they will merge into a yellowish orange if seen from dead ahead at any distance over about half a mile. The only way to ensure that the two colours will remain separate at their maximum range of visibility is to have separate lamps at least 6 feet apart, or more logically at the maximum beam of the vessel. With sailing boats that brings other problems, for it is difficult to find a place where lamps can be mounted with such separation, at an effective height, and yet be free from masking by a headsail. For that reason, the single bi-colour lamp, on the pulpit and forward of all sails, is probably the best answer, for the merging of the two colours is an effect limited to a viewer who is directly ahead.

In practice, many bi-colour lamps show nothing at all to a viewer who is dead ahead, nor even to one who is several degrees to either side, because a dividing bar between the glasses gets in the way. That was shown in tests made by the editor of *Yachting World* (*Yachting World, January 1971*), during which it was established that the coloured glass should meet edge to edge, and that there should be no opaque divider between them. This is really the most important single factor in currently available bi-colour lamps. In the long term the really important improvement will come from a properly designed optical system, using a reflector and a bulb whose filament is accurately positioned. But Heaven knows how long we shall have to wait for that.

Apart from the lamp-housing itself, the other very important consideration is the voltage of the current that reaches the bulb. The long cable run to the lamp, combined with the ordinary failings of lead-acid batteries means that the bulb which is designed to give its light output at 12 volts may be receiving current at one or two volts lower pressure. Almost every motorist will have observed the difference in the brightness of his headlamps when the engine is switched off and they are supplied by the battery alone. In fact, with engine running the voltage at the bulbs may be a little above 12, whereas with battery alone it will be a little below. For sailing craft, or wherever lights are to be run from batteries alone, one needs bulbs designed to run at, say, 10 volts, but I don't know where to buy them. All one can do in practice is to make sure that the voltage drop in the circuit is kept to the minimum. That means having wires of sufficiently heavy gauge. A cable amply thick to carry the required current with safety (i.e. without overheating) may reduce the pressure by as much as 2 volts in a 20-foot run. If the run can be halved, the drop will be halved too, which is something to bear in mind. Even a 'very heavy' cable, in ordinary boat-wiring terms, will give a voltage drop of between one third and one half of a volt for each 10 feet of run, so it is wise to err on the generous side when installing cables. (For those who are concerned to make all the calculations, there is a booklet available from Lucas-C.A.V. called *Marine Electrical Systems* which explains the whole thing.)

When running under power a boat must show a white light forward, and the bulb in this lamp can afford to be of a high wattage, for while the engine is running there should be an ample supply of current. The red and green lights, and the white stern light will in any case be brighter when the alternator is feeding into the battery, so the whole situation should be notably better than it is under sail.

Under the Collision Regulations a sailing vessel is permitted to carry additional red and green lights near her masthead. These optional lights are mounted one above the other (red uppermost) and sufficiently separated as to be clearly distinguished at 2 miles. *Each* light shows over the whole arc of the white forward steaming light – that's to say from $22\frac{1}{2}$ degrees abaft the beam on the one side to $22\frac{1}{2}$ degrees abaft the beam on the other. Just to make the point quite clear, each light covers the combined arc of the normal red and green lamps.

But these optional lights for sailing craft have never had much appeal for me. When one is short of current it seems to me more logical to concentrate the available supply into the obligatory lights – the usual ones – rather than to use it for two additional lamps, each of which will have to be 36w if it is to get anywhere near the 2 miles visibility prescribed. As has been said above, a sailing boat might very well have a 36w bulb in her bi-colour lamp, and a 12w bulb in her stern light, making a total of 48w. The red-over-green mast-lamps would add a further 72w to the load, and if that amount of current is going to be available then I feel sure that it could be better used.

Having done one's best to ensure that one's navigation lights are as bright as is feasible there is still one more shot in the locker – the' flare-up' light. This is a white light, and the use of the expression 'flare-up' in the Regulations implies a white pyrotechnic flare, or a cresset made of rags soaked in paraffin. White flares are carried by most yachtsmen for the purpose of drawing attention to themselves if the ordinary lights have not been seen, but there seems no reason why a flare-up light should not be electric. Thus a powerful torch whose intense beam can be directed toward a ship could meet the case. Even better, since one might not always know where to aim a beam, would be an all-round white masthead light of the greatest possible brilliance. This is not a lamp which is to be left burning but one to be flashed as necessary for short bursts. It really requires a masthead light with two bulbs in it (or possibly a double-filament bulb like the tail-and-brake lights of a motor car) but I don't know of any commercially-made unit for boats. It goes without saying that an owner can devise some form of bright white light for himself – the purpose after all is merely to attract attention, in the hope that the officer on the bridge will have his eye directed toward you and will thus notice your conventional lights.

Some owners carry an Aldis lamp for the purpose of attracting attention. This type of lamp has a narrow, pencil-like beam, and if it is to be seen by its intended recipient it must be carefully aimed, using the telescopic sight. If you are willing to go to the expense of such a lamp (about £15) it will certainly provide an excellent interpretation of the 'flare-up' light. It can also be used for signalling by Morse code – its originally intended purpose.

It is often said that you can attract attention by shining a torch on to the sails of a sailing boat. But the intensity of light reflected by a sail is far lower than the direct beam from the torch, always supposing that you can aim it effectively.

ON THE RADAR SCREEN

Officers on big ships nowadays depend greatly on what they can see on the radar screen, seeming often to prefer its information to what they might gather with their own eyes, even in good visibility. Taking into account the frequency of poor visibility in northern European waters, it is obvious that there will be many occasions when the fate of our vessel depends on the sort of reflection she gives to the radar set. That in turn leads to the inevitable conclusion that a small boat must carry a radar reflector.

Rather like 'cat's eyes' in the road, and other reflective signs, the radar reflector is so designed as to give a very strong echo. The use of plane surfaces at right-angles to each other so as to form three-faced corners has the effect of returning the signal back along the path whence it came. Any snooker-player can do the same thing with a ball, only in that case it is a two-dimensional problem only. Anybody with a ball and two walls making a right-angle with each other and with a level pavement can prove the three-dimensional case for himself. The important thing is that the angles shall be as nearly exact right-angles as possible – an error of one or two degrees is said to reduce the effectiveness as much as ten times. Furthermore, it is not correct to say that the echo will be equally strong in all directions. The strongest echo comes when the reflector is looking with one of its funnel-shaped mouths open toward the radar transmitter. That is why the gadget should be in the three-point suspension attitude, and not hung from a single corner with one plane horizontal and the other two vertical. But even in the correct attitude the echo is not uniform all the way round the horizon, so a certain amount of swinging may be helpful.

The size of the reflector is of crucial importance because the reflective performance is proportional to the fourth power of the linear dimension. That can be turned into a numerical example by taking a 12-inch reflector as a standard. If 3 inches are added, to make 15, then the effectiveness increases by 2½ times. Add a further 3 inches and the effect is doubled again. In other words, an 18-inch reflector is 5 times better than a

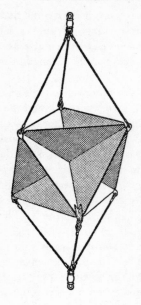

A radar reflector should be supported in the attitude shown here, and not with its planes parallel to the ground or upright. This is sometimes called the 'three point suspension' attitude, the reason for which should be clear from the drawing.

12-inch. The rapid change of reflective power with size means that there is a fairly clear change-over point between a reflector which is too small, and one which is big enough. In my opinion that comes at a size of 16 to 18 inches. Incidentally, it is the diagonal measure that is usually quoted by chandlers and manufacturers, and 16 to 18 inches would correspond to a side of about 11 to 13 inches. If you can go 2 or 3 inches bigger then I think you can expect to give a signal that will make you look like a large ship.

The smaller reflector may give an adequate signal on a calm day, and when all the circumstances are favourable. But when the weather is rough the operator on a ship may use the control to suppress the clutter of echoes coming from the seas themselves. A weak echo, coming from a small reflector low down in the waves, is likely to be lost in the process. In short one needs the largest practicable reflector, carried as high as possible. Subtle arguments can be put forward to show that some particular height is better than the masthead, but they ignore heeling and pitching and depend on special and rather hypothetical considerations.

The actual mounting of the thing presents practical problems which can be solved only in relation to one's own boat. A good look around at other people's solutions is perhaps the best starting point, but one also has to make a decision whether the reflector will be fixed aloft permanently, or hauled up on a halyard when needed. My own preference is for permanent fixing. A radar reflector is an awkward thing to stow – it really must be dismantled and folded flat – and it is a nuisance to re-assemble and haul aloft. Heavy rain, sea fog, or a passage that unexpectedly extends after daylight hours may call for its use at any time of the year, and on many such occasions the need to hoist the reflector will coincide with other worries such as heavy weather, difficult pilotage and so forth. In such conditions one could easily decide that it is too much bother ... and so be without the reflector when it was most needed.

FOG-HORNS

Little boats should be seen, especially so because they are most unlikely to be heard. In bad visibility sound signals are to be made by horn or by bell, according to the Collision Regulations. Such signals may be heard by the crews of other sailing craft, but it is quite unrealistic to suppose that they would be heard by the officers of large ships, ploughing confidently along on radar watch. As far as I know, the best fog-horns available for boats are the costly and unwieldy plunger-operated type, and even they have small chance of being heard on the bridge of a ship in sufficient time for her to take avoiding action. Their size is much against them and they are a rarity on family cruising boats. Far more common are the little aerosol canisters, but they are really too feeble to have much value as fog-horns, except between one small boat and another. Never the less, such a horn can be useful on board as a means of signalling one's manoeuvring intentions in accordance with the Collision Regulations (one blast, *turning to starboard*; two, *to port*; three, *astern*; five, '*what the devil's going on?*')

Motor craft, with a plentiful supply of electrical power can get powerful horns, of course. But for sailing craft the problem really lies with the inventors; just as there is a need to design and produce more efficient navigation lights, so there is a need for some kind of electronic hooter. A transistor radio on the beach seems to make a pretty loud noise, so surely something *useful* could be done with a circuit and a loudspeaker?

Indeed, the Tannoy loud-hailer has an oscillator which generates a hooter tone, and something along these lines may be the best answer. Even so, I doubt if the answer lies in sound signals at all. Little boats are not likely to be heard, and their best way of making their presence known is to be seen, either by reason of their lights, or by use of a radar reflector.

CROSSING THE SHIPPING LANES

A small craft will try as far as possible to keep clear of ships, and in coastal waters, estuaries and similar areas that can be done by holding to shoal water as far as possible. On the open sea there is no such possibility, but it is useful to know that commercial ships tend to take the shortest route from one point to the next. Often the 'points' are headlands, islands or other turning landmarks – places like Land's End, the Scilly Isles, the North Foreland and so forth. Thus, and with the help of *Reed's Almanac*, it is possible to get an idea of the shipping lanes where the danger of being run down is highest. *Reed's* will also show the special 'traffic separation' routes which are coming into use in congested waters. These special zones were made necessary because the world's shipping tends to take the shortest possible route between headlands, so that such points tend to be places where ships meet, going in opposite directions! There are also places like the Dover Straits where the navigable channels are narrow, in big-ship terms.

The traffic separation rules will not really be applicable to small craft, though it is important to have knowledge of what the big ships may be expected to do. As far as possible, the skipper of a small craft will tend to keep out of the shipping lanes. It is often said that it is best to work into shallow inshore waters, but although that has obvious merits it cannot be laid down as a standard policy. It may be just as easy to avoid shipping by going a little farther offshore, bearing in mind the tendency for ships to take the shortest routes. And farther offshore may be the better place for other reasons: the water may be less disturbed, overfalls may be avoided, and the risk of being embayed is eliminated. For example, when making slow progress against the tide off Portland Bill and its race, I have preferred to stand off about 12 miles, leaving the shipping en route between the two headlands of Start Point and St. Catherines to pass to the north. To try to keep *inshore* of those ships would have put me nearer to the race than I cared to go.

Nevertheless, many owners of small craft will be coasting for much of the time, and will quite naturally find themselves inshore of the shipping lanes. On those occasions when the lanes cannot be avoided, I think it best to try to sail *across* a lane rather than along it. Once across, one is fairly free of the threat until the next lane, and the crossing is most quickly done if it is as near to a right-angle as possible. On the other hand, to sail *along* a track frequented by ships is to expose oneself to the risk for the maximum of time. It is especially dangerous because the higher speed of the ships poses a threat from astern, a quarter in which it is not always easy to keep a good look-out.

A long, oblique crossing is also very trying, though it must sometimes be made of necessity. Indeed, the fact that a meeting with a ship may happen at any angle, and at a variety of speeds makes it impracticable to lay down any simple rules of behaviour. The actual right-of-way rules themselves must be known by every seagoing skipper of course (they are summarised at the end of this chapter), and there are also sound principles dictating the correct manoeuvres to avoid a collision in certain situations. But the fact is that big ships cannot always be relied upon to behave as they should, even when meeting another ship of their own fighting weight. Anyone who is skippering a very small boat may therefore be quite right to assume the worst and take evasive action, even when the bigger vessel *should* give way. It is equally a fact that a further danger is created when a small boat takes avoiding action in a situation where it is her right to stand on.

Consider a simple case, where you are proceeding under power and crossing a shipping lane more or less at a right-angle. Three miles or so out on your port hand you see a ship. At this stage you cannot be sure how your relative courses are shaping, but you are on her starboard hand, and it is therefore her duty to give way.

You take a bearing on her with the hand compass, and another a few minutes later: then a third. Because there is no change of bearing you know that you are indeed on a collision course, but you fear that she may not have seen you, or that for some other reason she may not yield. Rather than stand on your rights, you turn to port with the object of passing astern of her. If you aim your stem at her stern, you think, it cannot be long before she will pass ahead of you. But what if her master has at more or less the same time ordered a change of helm so that *he* will pass astern of *you?* In a moment or two you will see that great hull swinging her bow toward you, and realise that it would have been far better if you had stood on your course.

In fact the Collision Regulations instruct that the right-of-way vessel should hold her course. It is the logical thing – the necessary thing if the give-way vessel is to be able to plan her manoeuvre properly. When two gentlemen dither at a door and neither knows who is to have precedence they may collide, but a lady has precedence and both she and the gentleman know it.

Unfortunately the Collision Regulations are not always strictly followed in real life. I have it on the authority of several ships' officers, as well as some very experienced Trinity House pilots, that some commercial ships sailing up the English Channel have in recent years adopted the attitude that they are on the 'main road', and that north-south traffic crossing the Channel is on the 'minor road'. The fact that cross-Channel ferries and other commercial ships have experienced that behaviour suggests that we who go in small boats must expect to meet it too. In consequence, it is not enough to take the easy line, set out the Regulations and then urge all small craft to obey them. If one is realistic one must admit that there are occasions when the skipper of a small right-of-way craft will yield at an early stage of the encounter, making clear that he yielded by a distinct change of course. If that is to be done, then it is important to do it early, while there is still plenty of clear space between the two craft.

Perhaps the most important thing of all is to be able to

establish in one's own mind whether the two craft are on a collision course or not. If a ship is steaming approximately toward you, it is usually not too hard to discern whether her two masts are in line, or whether they show that she is in fact angled slightly to one side or the other. It may also be possible to see down the length of her hull on one side, a clear indication that she is not directly 'aimed' at you. By night her two steaming lights, of which the after one is the higher, will allow you to judge the attitude of her masts. Furthermore, she cannot be directly in line if you can see either her port or her starboard light.

If you do decide that a ship is heading straight for you everything will depend on your own course. If you are crossing her course, then the situation should soon correct itself – she cannot continue to head for you unless she turns. But if you are headed directly toward or away from her the situation will demand action. If the two of you are approaching head-on, then each should change course to starboard, so that you pass port to port. If she is coming up astern of you then it is her duty to keep clear though, feeling rather small, you may try to scuttle out of the way yourself. If you are tempted, remember the risk that you may turn just as she turns, and that you may merely put yourself into the line of her new course.

This situation where the ship seems to be aiming straight at you is a special case, but a particularly frightening one for many people. A ship bows-on looks very menacing, but a collision is just as possible when the two vessels are following tracks which will cross. The problem then is to know whether they will arrive at the crossing point at the same moment of time – whether they are on a collision course. As most people know, that problem is solved by taking bearings of the other vessel with a hand compass. If her bearing remains constant then the two of you are on a collision course. If the bearing is changing then you will pass clear. Using a 360-degree compass scale, one can say that a vessel approaching on your starboard hand will pass clear ahead if the bearing value decreases, and astern if it increases. The reverse applies if he is approaching from port. This is really rather obvious, and perhaps unnecessary because one can see which way the bearing is swinging.

The constant-bearing rule applies in all cases, and it can be especially useful if you believe that the other vessel is turning in such a way as to cancel your own evading manoeuvre. In other words, having detected a collision-course situation, and having manoeuvred to avoid it, you can check that your manoeuvre is effective by continuing to take bearings.

One of the most disconcerting things about one's first encounters with ships is the very great difference in speed. They travel so much faster than the typical small yacht, moving at 4 or 5 knots, that one's expectations may be quite upset. A ship that, when first seen, seems so far away that you feel there must be plenty of time to cross ahead of her, rapidly comes up and passes ahead of you. This is a situation where reliance on the hand-compass for successive bearings is better than a guess. The owner of a fast power cruiser is in a much better situation, of course, since he may be able to outpace many merchant ships, and will certainly have the power to manoeuvre very effectively. But no small craft, fast or slow, should approach too near the stern of a ship moving at speed – her wash may be very steep-faced, and more than you bargained for.

If only one could be sure that big ships would *all* obey the rules and give way when they ought, or equally if one could be sure that they would never give way but always stand on regardless, it would all be very much simpler. As things stand, it seems that we who are in the small boats will usually give way without regard to the rules. If that is the decision then it had best be done early and clearly so that if there is anybody on watch on the ship he will know in good time.

THE RULE OF THE ROAD – A REMINDER

The Collision Regulations stipulate that manoeuvres to avoid collision should be positive, taken in ample time and with due regard to good seamanship. Among other things that means that bluffing or holding on till the last minute in the hope that the other chap will give way is ruled out.

The rules themselves stipulate:

1. *When two vessels under power meet head on, each shall turn to starboard so that they pass port to port.* (Effectively the rule corresponds to 'driving on the right'.)

2. *An overtaking vessel always keeps clear of the vessel she is overtaking.* (Always – a sailing boat overtaking a power boat must keep clear.)

3. *Power boats give way to sail, except as in item (2) above, or when the power vessel is very large and is restricted by the navigable channel.* (Don't sail your 5-tonner across the bows of a liner in Southampton Water; she can't give way.)

4. *When two power vessels are on a crossing course, with risk of collision, the vessel which has the other on her starboard hand must give way.* ('Give way' means slow down, or stop, or turn to pass astern of the other vessel.)

5. *When two sailing vessels are approaching with risk of collision, and if they have the wind on the same side, the windward boat must keep clear.*

   But if they have the wind on opposite sides, then it is the boat with the wind on the port side that must keep out of the way. (The rules specifically state that 'wind on the port side' shall be defined by the fact that the mainsail is on the starboard side. That has many subtle implications, and is worth some thought.)

What I have written above is my own distillation of the rules as they are at the time of writing. But not for the first time in my life I find myself writing a book at a time when the Collision Regulations are about to be changed. To try and give both the new and the old, and at a time when nobody yet knows when the new rules will come into force, would be altogether too complex. Fortunately, the new Regulations, insofar as manoeuvring is concerned, are not much different from the old. But they do emphasise the points I have made – that small craft must not hamper big ships whose freedom to manoeuvre is restricted by shallow water or narrow channels.

The forthcoming Regulations (which may have already come forth as you read this) do have some special and rather technical things to say about navigation lights that should be carried. You can find all the details in Reed's Almanac, in *The Small-Boat Skipper's Handbook* by Geoff Lewis, or by getting your own copy of the Regs from Her Majesty's Stationery Office. Just ask for the 'Collision Regulations'.

One last word. Take heart. If the new rules about lights seem a bit daunting, take special note of *Part E. Exemptions*, wherein you will see that a period of several years' grace is allowed before the new requirements should be put into effect.

12. Bags of Air Will
Keep You Up

PERSONAL BUOYANCY

On my shelf I have a book about dinghy sailing. It was published in 1952 and in the dozens of pictures of boats under sail I can find only one where the crew appears to be wearing any sort of buoyancy garment.

Indeed, the general use of buoyancy jackets and lifejackets is quite recent in sailing. They have been made necessary by the vast increase in the popularity of 'capsizable' dinghies, and from there they have spread their popularity to cruising boats. Not that most people on cruising boats wear them all the time, but most boats carry such things nowadays, whereas in the pre-war years I am pretty sure that most boats did *not*. At any rate those with which I was acquainted did not.

This is not to say that there is anything against the current trend. Obviously personal buoyancy has its uses. In capsizable dinghies it is virtually imperative that it be worn, not because the crew may not be able to swim, but because there are circumstances in which even able swimmers can become tired, injured, overpowered, or even entangled in their own rigging. And in cruising boats the availability of buoyancy waistcoats of some kind is a valuable asset, whether you are risking a run ashore in choppy weather in a too-tiny dinghy, or whether you are at sea in a really serious situation.

No, buoyancy aids are fine, but their newness lends per-

168

spective to some of the arguments that have flourished on the difference between a *buoyancy aid* on the one hand and a *lifejacket* on the other. It is natural that discussion should thrive when an idea is new and is still growing. The important thing is to assess what you need, and not to split hairs in debate.

It is unfortunately true that you need quite a large amount of bulk in a lifejacket in order to get the amount of buoyancy that will keep your head above water in a really bad sea. In my own view that bulk can of itself be a danger when one is working aboard a boat, as can the presence of straps and loops which may catch in parts of the boat or her rigging. In the same way, a harness and safety line can present the hazard of tripping over your own line. But nothing is perfect, so one weighs the pros against the cons. Most people will find a middle road, and avoid either the extreme which says *always* wear buoyancy when on board, or that which says *never*.

Now, as it happens, the opposing qualities of adequate buoyancy and minimum bulk can be resolved if one accepts that there are two principle categories of use for a buoyancy garment.

Use One is that of the dinghy sailor. He needs to wear his aid virtually all the time. Therefore it must not be too bulky. But he does not go far from the land, usually sails within reach of other people, and normally rights his boat and re-boards her in the event of a capsize. So for him a moderate amount of buoyancy in a compact garment is quite appropriate.

Use Two is that of the sea-going and cruising man, or the fisherman who goes several miles out with no other boat for company. Such people do not normally wear any buoyancy at all. Their boats stay right way up, and they have 'fences' around their decks. The crew may also wear harness, which dinghy sailors do not. The sea-going man wants *his* buoyancy garment to be available in case of dire emergency – when he may be parted from his boat, out of sight of land and in a place where help may not come for many hours. Obviously he needs the maximum buoyancy, and since he expects never to wear it and if he does wear it he will be jolly glad to do so, bulk is of relatively small importance.

It is easy to think of exceptions to this pattern. The sea-going man who does not have lifelines around his boat and fears that he might go overboard even in a calm sea and under a blue sky may decide that he wants to assist his own powers of swimming by always wearing a light buoyancy aid. Very sensible.

A dinghy sailor who sails the sturdy, 'old-fashioned' type of boat which he has never yet capsized and probably never will, may turn his nose up at a slender wear-all-the-time waistcoat, but may carry a fully-buoyant lifejacket on board in case of some extreme situation.

And where children are concerned it is a sensible rule that they shall wear buoyancy aids all the time. Aboard such a boat the adults will wear aids too (all the time), to show what the trade unionists call solidarity.

A racing-dinghy sailor, who may expect to go into the water from time to time, may also make longer passages away from the pack, and therefore feel that a full lifejacket is what he needs. On the other hand he may feel that its bulk would be an unacceptable hindrance in the business of righting the boat and climbing back in, even though some of the air *could* be let out. He might decide that he ought to have two buoyancy garments, one for his racing when he wants minimum buoyancy and maximum freedom, the other for his longer excursions.

Similarly a cruising-boat owner might feel that he ought to have a full-buoyancy lifejacket for every person on board, but that waistcoats with a moderate amount of buoyancy should also be available for trips ashore in the dinghy. Such trips are indeed more likely to lead to a dunking than years of sailing the sea in a bigger boat.

One argument that is often heard concerns the person who is knocked on the head by the boom and goes into the water *unconscious*. If anyone does fall into the water in that state then only the fullest amount of buoyancy is likely to save him. What one has to decide therefore is how likely such an event really is. Personally I have never come across a case of it, but it must happen sometimes, just as people fall downstairs sometimes. And by the same token one could wrap oneself in a padded mattress before going down stairs, just in case . . .

It seems to me that unconsciousness is more likely to ensue after the person has been in the water some time, from cold and shock. Everyone has to make up his own mind, according to his own view of the realities of the situation, and not according to anyone else's pet theories.

Having made up one's mind there is plenty of choice, and the choices are changing all the time as new manufacturers come into the business, or as established firms 'improve' their old products or introduce new ones. (I felt obliged to put 'improve' in quotation marks because I believe that in the modern world many so-called improvements are nothing more than the results of manufacturing economies or short-cuts.)

In practical terms the two broad categories of buoyancy aid and lifejacket can be identified (at the time of writing) with two groups of approved aid.

Aids approved by the Ship and Boatbuilders National Federation are of the lesser buoyancy type – *buoyancy aids* – giving at least 18 lb of positive buoyancy to the wearer. This is the type of thing that, for example, takes the form of a slim waistcoat lined with closed-cell foam pads. It is possible to stick knives through these pads without having any appreciable effect on the amount of buoyancy available. Others have a large number of separate air-filled plastic sachets, and here again local damage does not have much impact on the effectiveness of the garment.

Full lifejackets come into the categories approved by the Department of Trade and Industry (formerly the Board of Trade) and the British Standards Institution. These give 35 lb or more of buoyancy when fully inflated – and they usually are of the inflatable type, though some have a certain amount of permanent buoyancy in the form of foam or the like. In this category one has real lifesavers, designed specifically to hold the head clear of the water, for which purpose they have a good-sized buoyancy chamber behind the wearer's neck.

Among these lifejackets of high buoyancy are some which inflate automatically. These are the ones, as the jokers say, about which there are never any complaints – if the thing fails the wearer is not likely to be in a position to complain. Some people would see an underlying truth in that sort of quip, for a real lifejacket may lie unnoticed for ten or twenty years before it is needed. Will the automatic device work after all that time? The maker may point out that it should have been sent back for regular servicing, and so it should. But will that happen?

A very practical garment is the one which has 18 or 20 lb of permanent built-in buoyancy, plus air bags which can be blown up by mouth to give 35 lb or more. It is, in effect, the two types of garment rolled into one.

That makes three broad types of garment from which one can choose. Unfortunately the matter becomes more complex when one has to consider the type of material from which the garment is made, whether it will tear easily, become brittle, or burn easily. (A fire on board may drive you into the water and is a very likely reason for resorting to a lifejacket.)

Then one has to consider comfort, ease of putting on and taking off, the reliability of fastenings. I never have much luck with zips in a salty atmosphere – even the plastic ones – but on the other hand tapes and strings can have their dangers.

It is indeed very hard to assess all the variables, of which price is one of the most important. I do believe that with the passage of time, and as the role of buoyancy garments becomes established, the boating public will resolve many of the questions on which so much hot air was expended in the sixties.

I also believe that for people who sail the bigger boats (not the dinghies) there is a good future for the waterproof jacket which embodies buoyancy *and* a safety harness. The need (hitherto) to put on a waterproof, and a lifejacket and a safety harness has been a deterrent to putting on any but the water-proof. When one can put on one jacket which does all three jobs there is very much less chance of being caught without harness or buoyancy in bad weather. Such garments have been available for some years, even as I write, but they are necessarily expensive, and many people already have a serviceable water-proof and a serviceable lifejacket so they only want to buy a harness. In other words, you need either to be in the position where you have none of the three items, or an excess of cash.

Children and infants present a special problem because the younger you are the greater is the weight of your head in relation to the rest of your body. And small children need more positive support for their heads than adults rather than less. To meet these two considerations in a lifejacket is not easy – it calls for a great deal of bulk. Nevertheless, there are a few firms which make lifejackets for children down to infant, and even baby size, while there are rather more who will provide buoyancy aids. Since children should wear some form of buoyancy for a large part of the time they are afloat, comfort and convenience are perhaps even more important than they are for adults. A good principle for all ages is that no aid is of any value if it is not worn; from which it follows that major factors in making a choice are such things as comfort and appearance and any other factors which tend to make the garment acceptable to the intended wearer.

LIFERAFTS

Perhaps the best of all buoyancy devices for the cruising family is an inflatable liferaft. Because exposure is the great killer at sea, a liferaft, with its canopy to give protection against wind, sun, rain and cold, is a real lifesaver. The lifejacket cannot compare.

Like the buoyancy garment that is now so popular, the inflated liferaft is a comparatively new thing, brought to the sea by way of the air and not really known until well after the Second World War. Sometime in the fifties it began to be generally recognised that an inflatable liferaft as carried by aeroplanes was a far more seaworthy device than the ship's lifeboat, ranged in davits on the deck with all her sisters. And as inflatables began to gain acceptance in the mercantile marine so they caught on in yachting circles where they were even more welcome because until their arrival it had not been possible for yachts to carry any sort of lifeboat. Size, of course, is the determining factor for a private yacht, and the owner has to be in the real millionaire class before he can hope to own a boat which is able to carry a second boat big enough to be of value in heavy weather.

Oddly enough there are still people who, presumably by analogy, have the vague idea that the 8-foot pram dinghy towed behind a 10-tonner, or inverted over her skylight, corresponds to the big ship's lifeboat. Unfortunately nothing could be farther from the truth. If two or three of the crew of the 10-tonner tried to row ashore in that pram in a choppy harbour they would have more than a fifty-fifty chance of filling her. In any sort of sea she would stand no chance at all, even with only two people in her. The inflatable raft, on the other hand, is extremely seaworthy and a far greater factor in the safety of sea-going crews than any lifejacket.

Many people who are familiar with rubber dinghies may suppose that a liferaft, in view of its more important role in life, will be made of heavier gauge and tougher material. But the reverse is the case, because the liferaft is expected to have an easier life than a dinghy, and also because it has to fold into the smallest possible space.

One result of this is that it really is essential for a liferaft to be returned every year to a qualified servicing base for overhaul. This will involve inflating the raft, to remove any creases, checking for leaks and corrosion, checking the automatic inflation gear and the ancillary equipment of the raft, and repacking. All in all it is a very thorough job and well worth the £20 or so that it will cost each year. But anybody who does not intend to have his liferaft serviced regularly and properly would be better advised not to buy one in the first place – he will most probably be wasting his money. And liferafts are not cheap. (At the time of writing they are priced at between £350 and £450 for a four-man size.)

The liferaft has certain qualities that no dinghy has, of which the chief is shelter for her occupants. Death at sea usually comes from exposure if drowning is avoided. The danger may be from cold, especially when a cold wind blows and clothes are wet, or it may be from excess heat. But the liferaft provides protection from the weather and allows people to stay alive for a virtually indefinite time, supposing that they have, first, water and, for longer periods, food.

The other characteristic of the liferaft is that she has stabilising water pockets – bags which hang beneath the raft

THE SMALL-BOAT SKIPPER'S SAFETY BOOK

and fill with water, whose weight acts as ballast to steady the craft. The protective canopy also keeps water out, other than what may come through the open look-out hatch, and that can be baled out. Every liferaft has a bailer and sponge among its other items of gear.

An inflatable dinghy cannot do the job of a liferaft, because it lacks the canopy and because its longer and relatively narrow shape does not give it the stability. But in spite of that, an inflatable dinghy is still far superior as a lifesaver to almost any rigid dinghy of the same size. And anyone who could rig an all-over canopy for an ordinary inflatable (I don't mean one of the beach-toy type), and stabilise her with a couple of buckets would be giving himself a much better chance than he would have in the water – even in the best lifejacket. The practical problem, of course, is to rig an effective all-over cover, because that is certainly not a thing which could be improvised in the moment of crisis when the boat is foundering and everybody is at 'panic stations'.

Ideally, any boat which is to cruise at sea should carry an automatically inflating liferaft, but they are expensive either to buy or to hire – and hiring for just the main two or three weeks' cruise of the year implies that you know when trouble will come, which cannot be known to mortal man. If a boat does not carry a liferaft (and that applies to most of us) then she should carry the next best thing, an inflatable dinghy in the fully- or half-inflated condition. It should have oars, bailer, air pump, flares and other desirable items lashed inside.

A liferaft proper will have at least two separately inflating compartments, thus minimising dangers due to leaks, and sometimes she will have a double-skinned inflatable floor as well. This reduces heat loss from the people sitting on the floor to the cold sea beneath them, though in the tropics such cooling may be welcomed. The raft is packed tightly into a rigid case or a valise of proofed material, from which it bursts like a butterfly from its chrysalis when it is inflated. Both the hull and the one or more arched tubes which support the canopy, are inflated automatically by carbon dioxide stored under pressure in a bottle.

Although inflation is automatic, it has to be started by a tug on the painter after the box or valise has been thrown into the water. The painter will be quite long, and its full length must be drawn out before the actuating tug can be made. Evidently, the end of the painter must be kept properly attached to the parent craft, and all on board must appreciate the need not to cast off the painter in the hurry of getting the raft into the water. Such a mistake could be easier than it sounds, especially on those boats where the liferaft is secured on deck by lashings which are intended to be *cut* in emergency. On the whole I dislike lashings for this purpose, if only because one always seems least likely to have a knife at hand when it is most needed. There are various metal slip-hooks, similar to the Sennhouse slip, which can be had from chandlers. Or secure lashings can be made from shock-cord, which can be stretched free, but the cord does not last very well, and it would probably need to be renewed every year.

Although liferafts are intended to be stowed on deck, and are therefore supplied in supposed watertight packings, those which I have seen in the workshops for their winter overhaul often show signs that water has penetrated – especially into the valise-packed types. Therefore I think that it is worth while to protect a rather costly investment with an additional cover – a simple piece of waterproof cloth with eyelets along its edges may serve also to hold the pack into its seating, especially if shock-cord is used to hold the cover down.

In positioning a liferaft on deck one must give thought to the need to get it clear quickly. Actually the thought should have been given by the designer of the boat in the early stages of the boat's conception, but that is rarely done and liferaft stowage is usually an all-too-obvious afterthought.

A liferaft forms its own fender, and it can be brought close alongside the parent boat for boarding without risk of harm to either craft or even to a person who might find himself nipped between them. If for any reason the raft cannot be brought alongside, the crew will have to swim to her and one assumes that they will be wearing some kind of buoyancy and harness too. The clip of the harness line can be made on to the liferaft painter for security, but even though the transfer is accomplished safely it is going to mean wet clothes. That is a bad start to what may be a prolonged attempt at survival.

The various liferaft makers provide slightly different packs of gear in their rafts. All have leak stoppers, bellows for topping up, a knife, bailer, sponge and instructions, but not all have distress flares and tins of drinking water. Although I have never had to use a liferaft in anger, I would think that these last two items are *essentials*. To have escaped from a sinking boat, say, and be safely in the raft but unable to attract attention seems an unthinkable prospect. And drinking water . . . the salt sea makes one thirsty, and any emergency or worry results in a dry mouth, which is a minor irritation perhaps, but not to be endured unnecessarily. And after twelve hours or a day, lack of water is going to become more than a minor irritation.

One possible solution, if one finds oneself facing the dilemma of a liferaft that seems right in all respects other than her provisioning, is to make up one's own 'panic bag'. This can have water, seasick pills, some first-aid gear, flares, a torch and other necessaries. It will of course have to be remembered by somebody, but that can be made easier if it is stowed under the extra waterproof cover I have suggested for the boxed raft on deck.

Just as when a big ship is abandoned the officers will load into the lifeboat blankets, flares, torches, and such other useful things as they may have time to take, so there is no reason why an inflatable raft should not be loaded with a few 'comforts', if there is time to do it, and up to a sensible limit of weight.

One item in the stores list of every liferaft is the booklet of survival instruction, which covers subjects such as conservation of body water, first aid, basic navigation and so forth. But instructions inside the raft will not avail for the situation where it inflates upside down, as occasionally happens. In that case there is nothing to do but the obvious – get into the water and heave the thing over by the handlines fitted for the purpose to the underside.

It is an unpleasant thought, but there are always balks of timber and other heavy objects floating awash in the sea – especially around populated coasts and near commercial ports. A collision with one of these almost invisible battering rams can make such a hole in a boat that she may sink very rapidly. I know one experienced yachtsman who had such an experience and his most sober estimate of the time his boat took to sink was between two and three minutes.

In a circumstance such as that a well-cared-for liferaft, properly stowed and ready for action, is probably the only hope. But even then it could prove useless if those on board have not mentally rehearsed themselves in its use.

To have a well-maintained liferaft on board gives a great sense of security, and is especially heartening to the father-cum-skipper who often feels his responsibility to his family-crew more keenly than they may realise. But although this is a really valuable piece of safety gear, one should not suppose that a day, or even a few hours, spent in a liferaft will be any sort of pleasure trip. The thing will probably save your lives, but in any sort of sea she is likely to make all on board feel seasick, which is one good reason why a supply of anti-sickness pills should be one of the items in the panic bag.

It may be thought that by concentrating in liferafts I am not allowing for the possibility that a leak may be stopped. Certainly it may, but only if it is a small one and if it is accessible. All manner of things may be used to stop a leak, and one of the simplest *may* be to trim the ship so that the damaged part lifts out of the water. I know one case of a boat on the Norfolk Broads which hit a floating balk with a resounding bang. Those on board felt sure that some damage must have been done, but there was no sign of rising water in the bilges so they carried on and forgot all about it. But in the early hours of the morning somebody awoke to find the cabin a foot deep in water.

The hull *had* been damaged but just above the waterline – at least while the crew were all aft in the cockpit. But with their weight distributed more forward in the boat at bedtime the crack was brought just below the waterline.

If one can get at a hole or crack it can be stuffed with rags or a cushion, or it can have a piece of plywood nailed over it or wedged in place. The difficulty is usually one of access, and since furnishings may have to be ripped away in a hurry, some experienced owners claim that a jemmy and an axe are essential tools aboard a sea-going boat.

Even if a leak can be staunched, or if it is by nature a slight leak, then the security of the boat will depend on the effectiveness of the bilge pumps. As I have said in an earlier chapter any boat which is above the size where bailers can be used effectively, should have two bilge pumps. They must be fitted with strainers so that they cannot become clogged, and if they are muscle-powered then they should be placed so that people can work while sitting down. Several hours of hard pumping may be needed, and that will not be possible in a stooping or crouched position.

Nowadays most boats have an engine – even sailing cruisers have an auxiliary – and in that case some form of powered pump makes a good mate for a hand pump. It may be driven mechanically from the engine or electrically from the battery – a fully immersible electric pump of good quality can be had for £20 to £40, and its special attraction is that it can be set to pump while crew members handle the boat, try to locate the leak, or do whatever is necessary.

13. Not Entirely On
Your Own

Setting out in a small boat one can feel very much alone, and it is indeed true that self-reliance must be the rule. That is the great difference between the cruising or pottering family and the racing folk who go out as a group and usually have a safety boat in attendance.

THE COASTGUARD AND THE CG 66

But around Britain's coasts you are not so much alone as it may seem, for there is a professional service devoted to watching those who go on the sea – Her Majesty's Coastguard. And the Coastguard does not merely watch – it has the responsibility for organising and directing rescue efforts when they are needed.

Some people think that the Coastguard are there to prevent smuggling – that they are the 'Revenue men' of the modern day, but although the service had its origins in Customs and Excise work, for the past fifty years it has been primarily concerned with the saving of life, and to some extent with the salvaging of wrecks. Their role is epitomised in the term Coastguard Rescue Headquarters (usually CRHQ) which is the name given to the principal station of each of the thirty-one Coastguard Districts around our shores. Each CRHQ is the principal reporting centre for its district, and is also an active watching station, keeping continuous look-out. There are also intermediate look-out stations, some of which keep constant watch, while others are normally manned only in daylight, but also at night when sea conditions are bad.

The service has about 550 permanent officers and men, but it is backed by the Coastguard Auxiliary Service – volunteers, who numbered around seven thousand at the last count. In short the service has the man-power to tackle such tasks as arise, and they are in fact many and varied. They may involve the rescue of people or animals perched on cliff ledges, or the more obvious rescue of seamen by breeches buoy. One thing the service seems always to be able to provide is initiative and ingenuity in tackling any lifesaving problem that may arise.

To yachtsmen the most important role of the Coastguard is the co-ordination of sea rescue services, which is indeed the main function of the service. If one sees a boat in distress the correct procedure is to dial 999 and ask for the Coastguard. You may think that a helicopter is needed, or an ambulance or a lifeboat, but the quickest and most effective way to bring professional help to bear is by ringing the CRHQ, which is what the telephone operator will give you. That is the centre which is in touch with all the relevant services, and it has the necessary communications links to call upon aircraft of the RAF, boats of the RNLI, ships of the RN, merchant ships at sea, or any other appropriate form of help.

An incident in the summer of 1969 when a man attempted to sail a *Mirror* dinghy the thirty-five sea miles from Newlyn in Cornwall to the Scilly Isles shows the complexity of a full-scale search. On that occasion tragedy ensued, for the dinghy was ultimately picked up in a damaged state which suggested that she might have been struck by another vessel, or perhaps dashed on the rocks. Nobody will now know what happened, but that does not detract from the efforts made on behalf of that lone helmsman.

He was in fact 'on a CG 66' as the saying goes. That's to say he had asked for Coastguard surveillance, and had completed a form CG 66, or had telephoned the nearest CRHQ where one of the staff would have completed it for him. This form records details of the yacht, her appearance, the number of crew on board, her destination, and her proposed times of departure and arrival. If she is coasting, each station will record her passage and pass details along to the next. If she does not arrive at her destination at a reasonable time, *or if the skipper forgets to report her safe arrival*, a search will be started. The italics should speak for themselves, but it is a fact that every year people turn out in to the cold night to search for crews who are snug in some bar.

Well, as I say, this chap bound for the Scillies had got himself on a CG 66. His boat was seen to leave and was watched until she disappeared into the haze, about five or six miles out. It was then 10.30 a.m. No great anxiety was felt when she did did not reach the Scillies that evening, for the winds were light and it was to be expected that she would make slow progress. Nevertheless, the CG asked the Land's End group of light-vessels if she had been seen, and the answer was 'no'. It was then arranged that a search would be made from the Scillies if she had not arrived by next morning. By seven o'clock that search was under way, and the RNLI had been given preliminary warning that they might be needed.

Within the next hour the Land's End group of lightvessels was warned of the non-arrival of the dinghy, so was *Scillonia*, the ship on the regular Scillies-mainland run. So, too, were the British European Airways Helicopter Unit which flies over the route, and the local trawler fleet. A bit later a harbourmaster down the coast reported that an incoming yacht had seen the *Mirror* for a few minutes in the haze, and that she seemed headed for Sennen. But Sennen reported that she had not gone there, nor had she popped into other harbours along the coast, all of which were checked.

At 9.43 a.m. a general broadcast to shipping was made from Land's End Radio, and the French authorities were asked to alert their trawler fleet by radio from Brest. At 12.30 a helicopter passenger said he had seen a dinghy that might have been the *Mirror*, and soon the St. Mary's lifeboat was out searching, while the inflatable Inshore Rescue Boat was searching the smaller, uninhabited isles of the Scillies, and Naval helicopters on exercise in the area were keeping a lookout too. Meanwhile harbours on the Cornish coasts were rechecked and some of the less likely ones were included this time. By the afternoon a Shackleton of the R.A.F. was out searching, and the search was extended to the Northern Cornish coast just in case ... Reports of various possible sightings were investigated, but nothing positive had been found by nightfall, when the search had to be called off.

It was at about 8.30 on the following morning that the empty but damaged dinghy was picked up off Gurnard's Head right round on the north side of Cornwall.

A story such as this, sad though it is, does show the scale of search that is required when a boat goes missing. Earlier the same year a vessel had reported by radio that she was aground near the Lizard light. After a long search involving three lifeboats and eight shore parties it turned out that she was in fact at Trevose Head, 50 miles farther north than her master had supposed. That was a merchant ship, not on a CG 66, but it underlines the difficulties of the searchers. So once again, if resort is had to the CG 66 procedure it is absolutely essential to report on arrival, especially if there has been a change of plan and you are not where you planned to be. Nobody wants to set in motion such large-scale searches without need.

SIGNALLING FOR HELP

A boat which is herself in trouble cannot dial 999, and the majority of us (who have no radio-transmitting equipment on board) must make our distress known by one of the other internationally agreed and understood signals. In many cases, of course, a watching coastguard may already have seen that your boat is in difficulty or danger, but you would not know of that, and even if you suspected it there would still be good reason to use distress signals as confirmation.

A coastguard or a seaman will recognise the agreed signals, of course, but an ordinary member of the public would react to only a few of them, and even then one must hope that he would know the right thing to do. Most people seem to tell the police, who *do* know that the CRHQ must be told. In practice the message gets through pretty swiftly, hundreds of times every year.

Let us look at the distress signals, starting with the one which 'every schoolboy knows' – the Red Ensign flying upside-down. Now although this is perhaps the one signal which almost everybody would interpret as a sign of distress, it so happens that it is *not* one of the internationally agreed signals. Presumably that is because some national ensigns look much the same either way up, or perhaps some governments are excessively sensitive about the thought of anyone seeing their national emblem upside-down. Nonetheless in British waters one can assume that an inverted ensign *would* alert most people if they noticed it, and certainly a coastguard.

The official signals are eleven in number, including one which can be sent only by radiotelephone. Still that leaves ten other methods available. (There is also the radiotelegraph alarm signal and the radiotelephone alarm signal, but these require equipment rather too sophisticated for ordinary private boat owners, and can be ignored for our purposes.)

I will list here the distress signals as described in the official words, with the preamble. For those who are interested they form Rule 31 of the Regulations for Preventing Collisions at Sea which is Annexe B to the International Convention for the Safety of Life at Sea. After giving the official wording I will enlarge somewhat on some aspects of the signals.

RULE 31

Distress Signals

(a) When a vessel or seaplane on the water is in distress and requires assistance from other vessels or from the shore, the following shall be the signals to be used or displayed by her, either together or separately, namely:

 (i) A gun or other explosive signal fired at intervals of about a minute.

 (ii) A continuous sounding with any fog signalling apparatus.

 (iii) Rockets or shells, throwing red stars fired one at a time at short intervals.

 (iv) A signal made by radiotelegraphy or by any other signalling method consisting of the group . . . — — — . . . in the Morse Code.

 (v) A signal sent by radiotelephone consisting of the spoken word 'Mayday'.

 (vi) The International Code Signal of distress indicated by N C.

 (vii) A signal consisting of a square flag having above or below it a ball or anything resembling a ball.

(viii) Flames on the vessel (as from a burning tar barrel, oil barrel, etc.).

 (ix) A rocket parachute flare or a hand flare showing a red light.

  (x) A smoke signal giving off a volume of orange-coloured smoke.

 (xi) Slowly and repeatedly raising and lowering arms outstretched to each side.

Then follows a note on the radiotelegraph and radiotelephone alarm signals which I have mentioned, and that is followed by:

(b) The use of any of the foregoing signals except for the purpose of indicating that a vessel or seaplane is in distress, and the use of any signals that may be confused with any of the above signals, is prohibited.

Well those are the actual words used in the English text of the Convention. But I hope that I may be excused for thinking that they will bear a little amplification.

Item (i), the gun or other explosive signal could easily be used by any of us *if* we happen to have a gun on board! But for the most part it seems of little use to the ordinary law-abiding boat-owner.

Item (ii) is more likely to be useful to the likes of us, because we should have some kind of fog-hooter on board, even if it is only one of those aerosol squeakers. But if one is going to use such a thing at all then one might as well sound S O S while one is about it, rather than hoot away at random.

That brings us, out of order but perfectly naturally, to item (iv). This allows one to make the signal ... — — — ... (which is S O S, of course) by *any* means. In other words you can use a hooter, or flash it by torch, or paint it on the sails, or chalk it on a large piece of cardboard (if you happen to have chalk and cardboard handy . . .).

Again moving out of order, but quite sensibly, we come to the signal N C. One would normally expect this one to be signalled by means of the code flags representing letters N and C, though the signal can be made by any means available. In the International Code of Signals, N C has the meaning 'I am in distress and require immediate assistance'.

And in spite of the fact that it is not listed in the distress signals of the International Convention, you could also fly the single flag V, whose meaning in the International Code is *I require assistance*. V, like nearly all the other signals in the new Code, may be sent by any means, and is not limited to a flag.

The single letter W is important in this context. It may be sent by any means, and indicates *I require medical assistance*. There are situations in which a red flare or orange smoke might be shown at the same time as flag W. A watching coastguard or lifeboatman would then know a bit more about the nature of your trouble.

Now let's skip back to item (iii) and consider it in conjunction with item (ix) since they both concern types of red firework. Obviously the red parachute flare which rises to a height of about 1000 feet and burns for 30 or 40 seconds while it falls slowly, is visible at a far greater distance than a hand-held flare. Whether it is more likely to be noticed than the star-shell flare which (rather like a glorified Roman Candle) sends a number (usually five) of stars to a goodly altitude, is arguable. The star shells burn for only about five seconds each, but their movement, and the fact that the same thing happens five times is likely to attract attention.

The hand-held flare may be more useful than high altitude signals if there is dense low cloud, though even then a parachute flare will often reveal its presence by a diffused glow. The hand flare also has merit for the final homing stage of the approach of a rescue vessel or a helicopter, to pinpoint your position.

By day, the thing to use is the orange smoke signal of item (x). A flare or star shell can also be used, but in daylight such things are not so easily seen. (The position of the sun in relation to a possible observer is obviously important.)

Parachute flares, hand flares, star shells, and a combined hand flare which also sends out star shells are all available from yacht chandlers. So are white flares, which are not a signal of distress, but may be used to draw attention to your vessel, perhaps to make people notice that you are flying a signal. More on flares in a little while, but first let's look at item (vii) which is an easy one to improvise. The round shape may be above or below the square shape, and it might be a cushion above or below a shirt or any odd bit of canvas. Indeed, one *ought* to carry on board a black ball to be displayed when lying at anchor, and although the ball is in fact no more than two black discs of plywood which can be slotted together at right-angles, most of us seem to find it too much bother to carry the gear. But anybody who cares to make himself not only the 'at anchor' discs, but also a black rectangle, can be equipped with an official distress signal at minimum cost and trouble.

There is little that attracts me about item (viii). It may be feasible to light a barrel of oil on the deck of a large steel ship, but I can't see how one could arrange a good show of flames from a typical family cruiser without adding to one's predicament.

Orange smoke (x) is an important daylight signal. The colour is chosen because it shows up well against the sea, and it is a great help to searching aircraft and ships in daylight. I doubt if one can improvise *orange* smoke, so it simply means buying the smoke canisters from your chandlers' shop. On the other hand, if I had no orange smoke canisters on board, then I would certainly try to improvise black smoke, since a searcher would be likely to investigate its origin if he saw it. Oil-soaked rags, with some paraffin to get them started, would make pretty good smoke. Rubber, if available, would be a fruity addition. The practical problem would probably not be in finding the fuel, but in arranging the fire in a safe manner. One thinks of setting the stuff in a metal bucket and somehow floating it away from the boat on the end of a cord, but unless you are going to sacrifice a lifebelt to support the bucket, it would be difficult to keep it afloat and upright, especially if there were a sea running. It might be possible to make a raft of such wood as was available, and float the oil-soaked rags away on that. But an altogether more convenient smoke-generator is likely to be found in plastics materials. Expanded polystyrene, which is like synthetic white cork, and which is used for buoyancy and for packing instruments, burns very readily, makes black smoke, and floats while it burns.

We have some foam-filled cushions on our boat, and by sacrificing a small scrap of the material I have found that it too will burn freely, making a good smoke. Other ideas will come to mind – it is something that each skipper can think about when he is in a suitably gloomy frame of mind.

Far simpler is the business of flapping the arms up and down (xi). A useful one this, because it calls for no special equipment. The difficulty is that in times of emergency one very often wants to use one's arms for other purposes – that certainly was the case on the one occasion when I wanted to signal for help. I had a 'woman overboard', and apart from getting the boat about and steering back to her I wanted to alert one or the other of two boats in sight. One of them, manned by two fishermen, saw my birdlike flappings, which I had to make while I steered back, sick and horror-struck, toward my wife. While actually flapping I was standing on the after-deck and using my feet to control the tiller – a procedure that could be prolonged only for a minute, perhaps, because as I came nearer the spot I needed to get a more accurate control of the boat.

Was I not grateful to those chaps who knew enough to recognise that I was not just playing the fool or giving an imitation of a well-fed swan trying to take off!

I was left single-handed when my wife went in, and the merit of this simple distress signal is that it could be made without delay. Obviously, in such a situation one has no time to go and fetch flares or haul up a signal flag (Flag O, 'man overboard') or anything of that kind. Your whole attention is on the victim and the boat.

That little incident impressed upon my mind the duality of distress signals – the need to receive as well as to send. A pretty obvious thing, I suppose, though I reckon that in some popular sailing centres you might fly flag V all day long and most boat-owners would take not the least bit of notice. Yet if they wanted to signal that *they* were in trouble they would be quick enough to look for their code-book or check card and find that V means 'I require assistance'.

The same chaps would probably be caught out if somebody were to flash U at them (di di da), because they would not know that it means 'you are running into danger'.

There is something of a digression, but it is perhaps worth noting that three dots and a dash tell *you* that *he* is in some sort of trouble, whereas two dots and a dash imply that *he* sees some danger ahead for *you*. Lord Randolph Churchill made a too-often quoted comment about 'those damned dots', but just one dot can make a deal of difference. Truly it is as important to be able to decode as it is to encode.

Back to the distress signals, and only item (v) to be discussed. I have already commented that relatively few yachtsmen have radiotelephones, though the number is growing steadily year by year. Those who do own them must surely have given some thought to procedures, which are important in radio communications, so I will leave that subject alone. One form of radiotelephone that is less costly and avoids the installation problems of the full gear is the emergency-only type of equipment. This is permanently tuned to the radio-telephone distress frequency of 2182 kiloHertz. The Post Office radio stations and the Coastguard CRHQs around the British coast maintain a permanent watch on this frequency, and ships' radio officers are enjoined to keep loudspeaker watch on it when they are not specifically engaged in any other trans-missions or receptions. Moreover, there are two radio silence periods of three minutes each in every hour – on the hour itself and at 30 minutes past. These are good times to send out a distress call if you have to. (For radiotelegraphy – Morse code – distress signals, the radio silence times are 15 and 45 minutes past each hour and the frequency to use is 500 kiloHertz.)

Those people who have radiotelephones of either the full-blown or the emergency-only type should already know that a distress call is started by saying *Mayday* three times in suc-cession. Then you give the name of your boat, her position as accurately as you are able to give it, the nature of the trouble, and the action you are taking.

Position information is obviously essential since you are not likely to be rescued if lifeboats and aircraft are searching in the wrong area. That is especially important with a radio distress call, for the range of even the emergency sets may be more than 150 miles in some conditions, and that opens up an extremely wide area of possible search.

One valuable thing that one can do with a radiotelephone is to report when assistance is no longer needed, or when help has arrived. That is something which cannot be done with flares, though it can be done by flying the flags E F, which have the meaning, 'S O S (or Mayday) has been cancelled'. Unfortunately, flags are visible only at relatively short distances, but like the other groups in the International Code, E F can be made in Morse code with a lamp or by any other means.

FLARE CARE

Although it ought to be known that fireworks of any kind should be stowed in the dry and not left to roll about where their cases can get damaged, not every boat owner seems to appreciate the point. People are usually reluctant to spend money on flares, just as they are with fire extinguishers, but in either case it is sensible to protect one's investment by proper care of the equipment after it has been bought. Flares will last many years if they are properly looked after. I know that they have an 'official' life of three years, but I myself have fired off flares that were more than ten years old, and I choose to look upon the three-year period as a purely formal one imposed on commercial shipping by the Department of Trade and Industry. I think it sensible to buy some new ones every four or five years, but I don't think it necessarily follows that the old ones should be destroyed, though a proportion of them can be fired as a test. A mixed bag of old and new flares is not such a bad thing, even if some of the old ones should fail to work when wanted.

On the other hand, there must come a time when old flares are discarded, and that is the opportunity to find out what it is like to fire one. Guy Fawkes night is the obvious time, and although you may see a warning on the case that pyrotechnics must be dumped at sea and not used for practice, I read that to imply practice *at sea*, where they would be taken for the real thing. Parachute flares can drop pieces of hot metal, so they should be used with care in populated areas. Each flare is dated

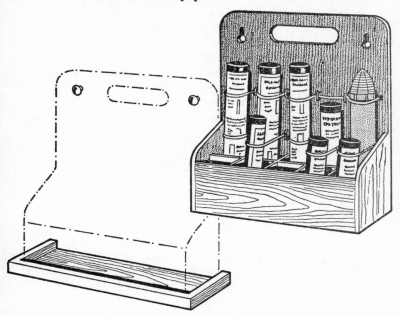

Flares may be kept in store for years before they are needed – perhaps in a hurry. A proper stowage like this has several merits. Flares are secure from damage or damp; are always in evidence; are stowed right way up and ready for use; and display their instructions, so that all members of the crew can easily remind themselves of firing procedure from time to time. Finally the whole thing can be picked up and taken aboard a liferaft or an inflatable dinghy. Dave Jenkins has shown a torch, which is a useful adjunct, but for the purpose of the drawing he has 're-moved' the plastic envelope in which each flare is normally sealed.

on its case, so it is easy enough to follow a plan of rotation, replacing a couple every year or so.

Flare stowage is not merely a matter of cosseting. The things must be easy to find, and quickly, whenever they may be wanted. Ideally they should be stowed in a special rack, where they are always in sight. It is not difficult to make a rack which ensures that the flares are visible and available to everybody on board, but also that they are stowed right way up. Although the firing of a flare is a simple procedure, the fact that it is done so rarely (and probably under stress or in the dark) makes it easy to bungle. One hears tales of people who have fired flares downward toward their own feet in the dark. Thus a stowage which presents the flare the right way up, and may also expose the instructions for anyone to peruse from time to time, is a step in the right direction.

Apart from that, it is obvious that one *ought* to make a conscious effort to study the firing procedure for each flare with the aim of being able to go through the drill without thinking if it should ever be necessary. There is no point in trying to detail the procedures for various flares here, but it is worth pointing out that nowadays they usually have some distinctive shape at one end which allows one to distinguish between top and bottom in the dark.

The actual firing of a flare involves no special risk – even the rocket parachutes go off without a bang and without recoil – but any firework may be a source of fire, and the odd spark or fragment of glowing case may cause trouble. Common sense dictates care, and that includes *not prodding or peering* into fireworks that have not gone off – or seem reluctant to go off. Some pyrotechnics take about 5 seconds between the pulling of the firing tab and the actual firing; so be patient. If after 10 seconds nothing has happened the only wise course is to chuck it overboard and try another.

Star shells, and parachute flares particularly should be aimed slightly downwind when firing. A rocket naturally tends to turn so as to head upwind, and if one begins by launching it in that direction it will turn to fly more or less horizontally and will not reach its proper height.

When and whether to use distress flares is a matter for judgement at the time. They must not be wasted in circumstances when there is no chance of their being seen. A parachute flare may be seen as far as 40 miles away on a clear night, star shells at about 10 miles, and a hand flare at about 5. The range of detection is likely to be decreased in daylight, but there are cases on record where hand flares have been seen at considerably more than 5 miles in daylight, so one cannot lay down any hard and fast rules. If one decides that it is worth sending up a parachute flare, then there is merit in the idea of sending a second one within about a minute. That will serve as confirmation to anyone who may have *thought* he saw something from the corner of his eye.

If one is near the shore then there is a fair chance that a distress signal will be acknowledged by the Coastguard. By day three bang-and-flash signals sent at intervals of about a minute, or the release of orange smoke, will indicate that your signal has been seen and that help is being organised. By night three white rocket stars at about one-minute intervals have the same welcome significance.

Even when one's call has been acknowledged, it is possible to give help to the searchers, as the following Coastguard report shows:

At 2102 on the 1 July Mr. Andrews, the Auxiliary Coastguard in Charge at Shingle Street [on the Suffolk coast] sighted red flares 1½ to 2 miles south-east of the look-out. He immediately answered the distress with three white star rockets. He then informed CRHQ Walton, who requested

Harwich lifeboat to launch. Shingle Street reported at 2118 having lost sight of a yacht, and the last bearing, 140° True, and course was given to the lifeboat. A Dutch yacht was then observed off the entrance to the River Ore, whose occupants were shouting as if to draw attention, but she then proceeded up the River Ore and it was considered unlikely to have been the craft concerned. At 2153 the lifeboat reported having seen a craft firing flares and that she was proceeding to her. A few minutes later the lifeboat reported having taken off a three-year-old child with·suspected pneumonia from the trimaran *Three Wishes*.

As it later turned out, the trimaran, all of whose occupants were Swedish, was on her way from Holland to England. But the wind was light and she had no fuel, and the parents of the sick child were getting worried about the delay in reaching medical attention. Thus the skipper decided to use his red flares, which were acknowledged. But the report shows that the lifeboat crew were having difficulty in finding the yacht, and it was sensible of the skipper to fire more red flares even after the acknowledgement. Evidently he used his judgement and fired his later flares after allowing a reasonable time for the lifeboat to be launched and to get under way.

Since there are so many internationally recognised ways of calling for help it seems pointless to try and devise private methods of one's own. Nevertheless I have seen various ideas put forward in books and magazines, and of these one can only say that if an accepted signal *cannot* be made, anything is perhaps better than nothing. The cartoonists always show shipwrecked mariners with shirt or trousers flying from the mast, and I suppose that many people would take that as a signal of distress, though it is normal practice to dry one's clothes in that way. I do have a record of at least one occasion when a RAF helicopter went out to a yacht whose owner was drying his trousers up the mast. Better safe than sorry, you might say, but it does seem rather a waste of time and money.

BEING RESCUED

That you can help searchers to help you is also shown by the example of two men whose cabin cruiser struck a submerged object in the Thames estuary one stormy November day. They fired several red flares, which were seen from the shore, but as their boat was sinking they took to their rubber liferaft in which they ultimately reached the Kentish shore, being helped in that direction by the northerly gale. On the way there they had been passed at a distance of only 50 yards by the lifeboat, which had not seen them (there were rough seas and snow squalls). There was also another boat out searching as well as patrols on shore. This is a case where hand flares would have paid off – the chaps in the raft shouted when they saw the lifeboat, but it was useless in that weather.

It is not possible to describe in advance all the possible actions that one might take to help rescuers – in an infinite variety of situations. But even the normal Sunday afternoon 'rescue' of a becalmed dinghy is often hampered because those on board have not bothered to prepare for towing while they have been waiting. Fenders can be got ready, and a heaving line with a monkey's paw or similar heavy knot at the end; everyone can get into lifejackets and harness; valuables and the ship's papers can be put into a bag. Evidently it is not enough just to collapse in a heap and await whatever God may send.

THE BREECHES BUOY

Broadly speaking, help may come in three ways – from the air, from the sea, or from the land. The third case implies that your vessel is ashore or on the rocks, and is likely to involve the use of some kind of line and perhaps of the breeches buoy. In each case active co-operation is required from those being rescued, and especially with the breeches buoy because those on board the distressed craft have to attach the lines at their end.

The Coastguard team begins by firing out the messenger line with a rocket. It is remarkable with what skill they seem to be able to fire their rockets so that the line falls across the vessel, but it can obviously call for more than one attempt.

When the messenger is across your vessel you signal 'OK' to the shore by waving your arm (with handkerchief or anything else that helps visibility) *vertically*. In all the procedures a horizontal wave indicates negatives, such as *no*, or *not yet*, or *not ready*. With an affirmative signal from the shore you can

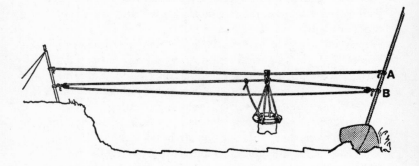

H.M. Coastguard have saved many lives with rocket line-throwing apparatus and the breeches buoy. A light line is fired over the ship by rocket, and those on board use it to haul out the tailblock (B) of the endless whip. This is made fast to the mast or a suitably high part of the structure. The shore party then uses the endless whip to send out the jackstay which must be attached at a higher point (A).

haul in on the messenger line, bringing aboard a block with an endless rope rove through it. This rope is the motive power for taking people ashore. The block has a rope tail which you must bend on to your mast, or some other strong point at a suitable height.

If you are on a boat with suitable mast a second line, the jackstay, will be sent out to you by means of the endless rope. This is the rope railway which is to support the breeches buoy, and it must therefore be attached higher up the mast than the tail-block. When it is sent out it will have a free end, and this should be made fast to the mast before the jackstay itself is un-bent from the endless rope – otherwise you will have difficulty in coping with the tension due to its weight and you might lose it.

On some boats, such as small motor cruisers, it may not be possible to find a higher point for the jackstay, and in that case the breeches buoy will be attached directly to the endless rope, and the journey will be made on that. In such a case, and indeed with any small craft, there is more chance that the passenger will dip into the water on the way ashore. But that is not significant because the *buoy* part of the breeches buoy is there to keep him from going under. A further safeguard is that the occupant will attach the clip of his safety harness to the sling of the breeches or to the endless rope – assuming that he is wearing a harness as he ought.

RESCUE BY HELICOPTER

The downdraught from a helicopter's main rotor is very severe, strong enough in fact to lay a small cruiser flat in the water if her sails are still set. Thus, a small cruiser or a dinghy which is being approached by rescue helicopter should get her sails stowed.

To lift people from a boat the helicopter sends down a

member of her crew on the end of a cable, so that he can help the victim into the harness and accompany him as they are winched up to the helicopter together. It is evidently very important that the cable shall not get foul of anything aboard the boat, and on sailing craft with much standing rigging it may not be practicable to lift people from the boat herself. In that case people may be lifted from a rubber dinghy or life-raft, streamed on a long painter from the parent vessel, or they may be lifted out of the water. This latter course implies that each person is wearing buoyancy, and it would be wise to keep a link with the boat by means of a long line, though it must be quickly detachable.

If the crew of the boat herself have no dinghy, liferaft nor lifejackets, the helicopter may lower an inflatable dinghy in which they will be able to float clear.

Two or three finer points: the helicopter chaps point out that you may get a slight electric shock when you make contact with the winch cable. It comes from the static charge picked up by the aircraft by friction with the air, and is of no significance. If you have to go into the water to be picked up, remove boots but not socks. And finally, when you are lifted by the winch to the aircraft door, take the passive part. The air crew will manoeuvre you into the cabin with far more skill than you could do it yourself – they've done it before.

RESCUE BY BOAT, AND THE SALVAGE-QUESTION

Rescue by another vessel may involve all permutations of sizes of craft and weather. It may simply be a case where a dinghy is taken in tow by one of the outboard-powered in-flatable boats of the RNLI Inshore Rescue Service, or it may be a matter of making desperate leaps from a wildly heaving motor cruiser to the boarding ladder of a large merchant ship.

In all the many possible situations it is seamanship that must be of primary importance. The handling of your own craft, her trimming for towing if she is a dinghy (including the raising of the centreboard of course), the preparation of fenders, and the choosing of the best moment to lay alongside if it is a big-ship encounter, the dealing with lines and so forth are all matters of boathandling. Nobody can foretell what will happen, and everything will depend on the ability of the skippers and crews of the two craft involved in handling their vessels. In short we are verging on another entire subject which calls for a book to itself.

But there is one aspect that sometimes causes concern – *salvage*. At some time or other we have all been told that if our boat is salvaged we, or our insurers, will be liable to pay a large fee to the salvor.

Most people would think that perfectly fair, but there are those frightening stories, 'Never use *their* warp, old boy, they'll be able to claim salvage if you do ... and above all, never let one of their chaps come aboard your boat ...'

And then there's the advice always to reach an agreed fee before accepting a tow, a concept which seems to me to ignore the realities of the situation. Negotiations over an office table have little in common with an exchange shouted across the wind and spray by a boat-owner who is wet, tired and probably frightened.

Like all legal matters this is one where it is risky for the layman to say very much, but as I understand it, there are certain basic points to be borne in mind as guidelines which may help one to fend off the occasional ruthless salvage-shark. But above all, I cannot help feeling that the principle objective must be to see one's vessel salved, and that legal arguments can wait till later.

As I understand it, there are certain principles which lie

beneath all the bar-side injunctions on the matter of salvage. In the first place salvage concerns property not people. The master of any British registered vessel is under an obligation to do everything he can to save life at sea. No charge can arise for doing that. On the other hand he is not under obligation to retrieve property, but if he does so voluntarily he can claim salvage, and the Admiralty Court may, after hearing what both sides have to say, make him an award.

To make a successful claim for salvage, the salvor must establish that the boat, or other property, was in danger. You can't just pluck a boat off her mooring and tow her ashore in triumph! Nor will a salvage claim stand where there is an ordinary commercial transaction – hence the advice to fix a price for a stated service before the salvor is allowed to act.

Whether or not the salved property was in danger is crucial to any legal wrangle over the salvage claim, and the fact will have to be decided upon such evidence as is available. If the owner of the rescued vessel has fired red distress signals there is an obvious inference that his craft was in some danger. If he was unable to pass a line to the salving vessel, or so weak or incompetent that he could not make a line fast, nor remain at his own helm, then the inference is even stronger.

Here one sees the underlying reason for all those warnings about letting chaps come aboard, and taking *their* lines. The crafty old fisherman who is claiming may point to the gale force wind, the nearness of the rocks, the inadequacy of your warp which forced him to use his own. In his view your boat was in extreme danger, and his reward should correspond. But you may be able to show that the wind was only Force 4, and that the rocks were fully 3 miles away. A good deal is going to depend on your behaviour, on the records of your log-book and any other evidence you can bring.

And one can see subtleties. You might run aground and

accept a tow from a passing boat. At the time you were in no danger, but if a fresh wind should spring up later in the day the salvor might be able to say that he had saved you from the bad pounding that you *would* have suffered had you stayed on the ground. Here again, the legal decision will be a matter of fact – whether the yacht was in danger, either imminent or future.

No salvage is payable if the boat is not saved. The *attempt* does not win the reward. It must be a successful attempt.

If the facts are that a vessel in *danger* was *successfully salved*, and that there was *no prior agreement* of a fee for the service, the value of the award will be based upon a number of considerations. Among them the value of the salved vessel and the degree of danger she was in; the value of the salvor's vessel and any danger she was in as a consequence of her service; any danger to the salvor's crew; and the time and expense involved to the salvor.

As I see it, this all boils down to the principle that if you need help you should try to ask for it as a competent, self-reliant skipper and crew, and not from your knees. At the same time one has to remember that there must be some 'salvage-sharks' in this wicked world who will offer the hand of friend-ship, such as the loan of a heavy anchor when yours is dragging in a gale, and later point out that their action was the saving of your vessel. Our protection, it seems is to reduce the kind offer of help to a sordid commercial level with a 'yes, I would like to hire that heavy anchor for a bit – will you accept a quid?' If such a contractual relationship is established a claim for salvage cannot stand.

In concluding this rather tawdry aspect of the noble business of rescue it is important to make clear the position of the crews of the Royal National Lifeboat Institution. These men will readily risk their lives to save ours, but they are under no obligation to save our property. If they do save property they are as much entitled to claim salvage as anybody else, and though it goes against the grain to seem to haggle with men who have come out to save your life, one should in principle try to agree a fee for any salvage service before it is done. For myself I rather doubt if I would feel like striking a hard bargain when *in extremis*. I hope never to put the matter to the test.

14. Last Look Round
Before Setting Sail

It was an introduction to sailing for my friend. We had had a pleasant enough morning and had anchored for lunch and a talk about sailing and the way in which he might take it up.

Now was the moment to get under way again. 'With wind and tide together,' I explained 'it will be easy to get the mainsail up . . .' and suiting the action to the words I gave a smart pull on the halyard and saw the rudder flick into the air and drop into the ebbing stream.

It's not really a safety story, I suppose, but it does serve to show that all manner of unexpected things can happen – and they *do*. In this case the mainsheet had taken a turn round the tiller, and the transom-hung rudder had no latch to prevent it lifting off its gudgeons. (We had no dinghy, but swimming with frog-feet, I eventually brought it back.)

Not everything can be foreseen, but one can make a regular practice of checking for fuel leaks, looking aloft at the rigging and making sure that shackle pins are tight, examining ropes for signs of wear, and so forth.

Sometimes it is the obvious things that are forgotten – warm clothes for example. Perhaps they are not so much forgotten as left behind deliberately, because conditions at the start of the day seem too balmy ever to change. But, as I have said in earlier chapters, coastal weather can change very rapidly, and there is also the possibility that you may be out longer than you expected. A minor trouble, such as an engine failure, a lost oar, a snapped halyard, something trivial in itself may delay your return till evening, or even until the weather changes quite definitely for the worse.

In an open boat it is not at all a bad thing to have a contingency plan for some kind of weather protection. A suitable piece of canvas can provide shelter for the crew, and it may even help to keep water out of the boat if the sea gets rough.

People need protection from cold and wet – they may also need protection from the sun for both skin and eyes. A first-aid kit is an obvious essential for the well-being of the human complement. Perhaps such things are obvious, but they can be overlooked, probably because they are not specifically 'boaty' items.

The specific safety gear that one carries depends to some extent on circumstances. In a sense, every component of the boat may be a 'safety' item, insofar as its proper working is necessary to the conduct of the ship. But there are some items that one can reasonably set aside in a special safety category. These include such things as lifebuoys and fire extinguishers, but they also include normal equipment such as an anchor and a compass, and a **radio** which can receive the shipping forecasts.

For a river boat, a **compass** is not a normal piece of equipment, and strangely enough some people who go to sea with the intention of anchoring a mile offshore for fishing also look on it as something rather special. But for anyone who goes on the sea, or even on a large inland loch, a compass seems to me to be an essential part of the gear, for (as I've remarked before) mist and rain can quickly reduce visibility to nil. Nor is it safe to assume that the boat will be so close to the shore that it will be possible to bring her in before the weather gets too thick.

What if the anchor cable parts, or the engine breaks down, or an oar is lost overboard? May she not find herself farther offshore than was ever intended? May she not be still at sea long after night has fallen?

A compass, fitted in some position where it is clear of ironwork, petrol cans, tinned food, bait-spades and the like, is a first requirement for any sea-going boat. It need not be a very expensive instrument, so long as the skipper locates it sensibly in the boat and takes the trouble to check its readings on known courses when the visibility is good. A second, handheld compass for taking bearings is valuable for collision-course problems (Chapter 11) as well as for navigation.

To check the compass implies the presence of a **chart**, and that too is a most desirable item on any sea-going boat. So, of course, is a **tide-table** and some guide to the set of the tidal streams. Whether that will be an Admiralty Tidal Atlas (which is not nearly so grand as it sounds – it is a slim pamphlet which costs only a few bob), or some pages torn out of an old copy of *Reed's*, or the insert sketches on a Stanford's chart, some knowledge of the set of the tide is essential. Not perhaps when things are going right, but vital when they begin to go wrong.

In bigger craft, which intend to cruise the sea all the above items will be on board in the ordinary way, and not merely as 'safety' gear. Charts will be more numerous, extending beyond the expected cruising range, just in case, and there will probably be a second compass. **Tidal atlases, pilot books,** *Reed's Almanac*, and a **leadline** or **echosounder** will also be carried as a matter of course. All of them have their safety implications.

For any craft an effective **anchor** and **cable** is a most important item. It may be the means of preventing a river cruiser from being swept down on to a bridge pier, or of holding a sea cruiser off a cruel shingle bank. Sea-going craft will normally have at least two anchors, and though only one of them may have chain cable, the skipper will have ample rope cable in reserve. I confess to carrying three anchors on board, each of them of a generous weight for our boat. Two of them have never so far been used (the same may be said of all the fire extinguishers) and that is something to be glad of. But in the past I have had to moor to two anchors in a gale, and it may happen again.

I have said a great deal about fire in an earlier chapter, and I admit that it *is* a tedious subject. One hardly need say that a well-equipped boat has a sufficient supply of **extinguishers**. But it should be added that one, two, or more **buckets** should also be at hand since it would be sad to find oneself with a burning boat, surrounded by millions of gallons of the finest extinguishant known to man, and nothing but your boots to collect it in!

In bigger craft several buckets would be needed in a fire, and each must have a **lanyard** attached, so that it can reach the water. That's not something that can be left until the heat's on. In a small open boat the bucket is also valuable as a high-speed bailer, though there must be a smaller **bailer** as well, and usually a **bilge pump**. Larger boats can benefit from having two pumps, and they should be properly installed with strainers to ensure that they cannot become clogged. Sooner or later one will become clogged, of course, which is one of the reasons why it is a good thing to have two.

Incidentally, in small craft, where the bucket can double for bailing and fire-fighting, a bilge pump may do the same. If it is portable it can be used to pump sea water *into* the boat if circumstances suggest that that is the right thing to do.

Good **lights**, so that you can be seen at night, and a **radar reflector** must also go on the list. These items have been discussed, in earlier chapters, but a point may be added concerning small craft under oars. They are not required to carry red and green lights, but must have a **torch** or **paraffin lamp** which must be 'exhibited in sufficient time to prevent collision'. If it were me that might be run down in a rowing boat I would take jolly good care to 'exhibit' a nice bright light in *plenty* of time to avoid that collision – not just *sufficient*.

A torch is also a valuable signalling device, as has been explained in Chapter 11, and will help other people to find you if it comes to it. But in addition to a torch, even the smallest open boat that goes to sea should carry some **red flares** and some **orange smoke** signals. And in this context I would mean 'sea' to include estuaries, and places like Plymouth Sound, say. In fact almost anywhere that is beyond shouting distance.

A **first-aid kit** for the people on board must obviously go on the list: and so must a **first-aid kit for the engine** that you hope will take you safely back to port. Just what either of these kits should contain will depend on the type of boat, the extent of her cruising and the type of engine. But there's no harm done if you have too much in the spares and repairs boxes. And if none of it is ever used, so much the better.

A separate **reserve of fuel** is, I think, a valuable safety item. Such a thing would certainly make a noticeable reduction in the number of lifeboat calls each year.

Where a boat is big enough a **lifebuoy** with 30 or more feet of floating line should be carried on board. In craft where space is too restricted a floating **quoit**, with line attached, can be the means of saving a man overboard. In bigger craft a couple of lifebuoys, *and* a quoit, *plus* **buoyant cushions** and similar items should also be available. And if a reasonably strong swimmer is normally numbered among the crew he should have a pair of **frog-feet** ready for use. These flippers make so great a difference to the power of a swimmer that I think it well worth the time that must be spent in putting them on. It is not time wasted, and with their aid a swimmer who can take a line to a victim in the water can be one of the most effective of all rescue devices.

On bigger craft, the **bathing ladder** is, I repeat, an essential item of safety equipment. The fact that a strong man can clamber back on board after a comfortable swim is not relevant to the sort of performance he might put up when weakened by cold and shock, and by his struggles with a rough sea.

On all boats there must be **lifejackets** (or buoyancy waist-coats) for all on board, and on sea-going cruisers there must be sufficient sets of **safety harness** for the deck watch at least. Some would say that every member of the crew should have his own harness, but I don't believe that that is strictly necessary, or that better ways cannot be found of spending the money. On the other hand, where money is no restraint then let there be harnesses for the maximum number of people ever likely to be aboard.

For bigger, sea-cruising craft only, a major item on the list is a proper inflatable **liferaft** of suitable size for the ship's complement, or a good quality **inflatable dinghy**. The life-raft will inflate automatically, but if a dinghy is substituted, it really should be kept inflated, though some people think it adequate to keep one of its two main compartments full and to deflate the other. That certainly eases the deck stowage problem, but it may be better to keep the boat fully inflated and to tow her astern – perhaps with two painters lifting her partly out of the water and up on to the stern of the mother ship. In any case, oars, bailers, pump and all the rest should be in the boat and tied there. Although the Department of Trade and Industry accepts the use of a rigid dinghy with permanently fitted buoyancy as a substitute for liferaft or inflatable dinghy, I cannot say that I would feel happy with that solution. To be effective as a lifeboat a rigid dinghy would have

BIBLIOGRAPHY

Bibliography is a grand word – too grand for the rather short list of books I have been able to compile on the specific subject of safety. But as I have tried to make clear throughout this book, safety in boats depends mainly on the power to imagine or foresee the kinds of trouble that may arise. And the best help for that, apart from experiencing a multiplicity of troubles oneself, is to read as widely as possible. Books on seamanship, and accounts of cruises and voyages, will always yield a point or two, sometimes more, to the mind that is alert to safety problems.

There are hundreds such books, but for anyone who does not quite know where to start, I have listed a few titles beyond those overtly devoted to safety.

SAFETY BOOKS

Lifeboat Handbook, George J. Bonwick, Maritime Press

Regulations for Preventing Collisions at Sea, Cmnd 1949, Her Majesty's Stationery Office

Safety Afloat, W. Zantvoort, Hollis & Carter

Safety in Small Craft, D. A. Rayner, Adlard Coles

Safety on Small Craft, Her Majesty's Stationery Office

Sea Wisdom for Small Craft, Hilary and K. J. Wickham, Stanley Paul

Survival at Sea – inflatable liferafts, Cmdr N. F. Keene, Maritime Press

GENERAL

All Seasons' Yachtsman, Peter Haward, Adlard Coles
At Home in Deep Waters, Bruce Fraser, Geo Newnes
Cruising Under Sail, Eric C. Hiscock, Oxford University Press
Heavy Weather Sailing, K. Adlard Coles, Adlard Coles
Pocket Cruisers, A New Approach, J. D. Sleightholme, Adlard Coles
Sea and Me, The, Humphrey Barton, Robert Ross
Small Boat Cruising, D. M. Desoutter, Faber & Faber

INDEX

217